Knee Pain

Effective Treatment to Speeding Up the Healing

(How I Proved My Doctors Wrong and Beat Chronic Knee Pain)

Sandra Maxwell

Published By **Oliver Leish**

Sandra Maxwell

Knee Pain: Effective Treatment to Speeding Up the Healing (How I Proved My Doctors Wrong and Beat Chronic Knee Pain)

ISBN 978-1-77485-544-7

Legal & Disclaimer

Table of contents

Introduction

Osteoarthritis (OA) can be described as an autoimmune disease of joints that has a major impact on people. It is a persistent and incurable disease. Edema, pain and stiffness are among the most frequent symptoms of this type of condition. As the illness progresses and progresses, symptoms like disabilities, problems in daily life and self-care, as well as chronic pain can manifest. Early-stage disease is characterised by changes to bone, synovium, cartilage and other joints, which do not always manifest. This is why patients are not aware that they suffer from osteoarthritis until condition has advanced and has become irreparable, as demonstrated by images. But, even though cartilage degeneration and loss are the primary causes of the process of developing osteoarthritis (OA) and provide some explanations for the shrinking of joint space as seen in x-rays tissues are affected. Numerous factors increase the risk of developing osteoarthritis (OA) but the precise pathways that lead to OA in individuals are not yet clear, leading to the reduction of treatment options. Therefore, people who are suffering from extreme pain and are unable perform work, provide for themselves, or walk could look into cell therapies for chronic pain disability, or a complete joint replacement.

Chapter 1: Guide To Knee Anatomy

The power of knowledge is in the mind. Don't they claim? Now, your strength is in understanding the problems in your knees which cause such discomfort and pain, as well as doing the things necessary for accelerate healing swiftly and efficiently. The best way to do this is to know the knees, prior to when all of the problems began.

You already recognize the knees are that mysterious, swollen lump between your legs between your calves and legs. In addition, you'll be aware that it bends in order to allow you to experience a variety of motion, however this may be the extent of your knowledge is. You aren't aware of the knee's mechanics and have never had to, up until the moment the knees started to cause you so much discomfort.

Let's make a change by starting right now.

In this section, I'll provide the fundamentals of the anatomy of knees in a manner that is simple to comprehend and is free of the type of jargon used in many knee-related textbooks seem to love. You will learn how your knee's structure is created and the causes of a knee injury.

Knee Anatomy Explained

Your knees are among the most vital joints of your body since they support your entire weight, and even more so if you jump, run or engage in certain activities. It's a hinge joint , referred to by medical terminology by the name synovial joint that lets you bend and stretch your leg, and experience the full range of motion.

The medical term used to describe your knee joint is the tibiofemoral joint.

Bones

It's where three bones join the Tibia (lower lower leg bone) as well as your the femur (thigh bone) and patella (kneecap). Imagine it as two bones that meet in the middle, with round bones over the point where they meet.

Meniscus

In between the bones lies the tough tissue, known as the meniscus. It is a shock-absorbing device and keeps the bones' ends from colliding and thereby protecting your bones from suffering and injury.

Cartilage

The bones' ends are covered by cartilage, which allows them to move easily over one another and protects against damage.

Joint Capsule

The bones that are located over them have the joint capsule, which protects the joint and gives durability and lubrication. Synovial fluid is made within this capsule, which feeds and lubricates joints.

Ligaments

Ligaments are affixed to this capsule to join everything and ensure that everything is perfect in alignment.

We spend the majority of our lives ignoring the fact that knees function so well However, just one issue in one place can lead to problems throughout your knee and alter the quality of your life.

In the next chapters in the chapters to follow, we'll begin to look more closely at what causes issues, the conditions they cause and the best way to go in order to fix these issues.

Let's first look at the reasons that could be causing knee discomfort.

Chapter 2: Diagnosing Knee-Related Problems

As you've seen in the previous chapter we tend to take for granted the amount of movement and motion our knees permit us to enjoy. This is until something goes wrong.

A lot of people struggle with chronic knee pain. They are thinking that the options available to them are limited , so they attempt to grin and bear it' getting some temporary relief, soon they notice that familiar sensation of a twinge reappearing. They are then afflicted with the same debilitating pain repeatedly.

This is a complete nonsense. I believe that everyone should have knees that are healthy and live a fuller living experience. I also believe there is always a solution regardless of how it takes to find it, and regardless of the advice of your doctor. suggest.

If you are determined to get rid of your knee pain completely You'll have to find what is causing the issue and identify the cause. You can treat only the symptoms, without considering the root of the issue and you'll never beat your pain. Life is too short for you to be unable to walk with no discomfort or pain.

There are three types of categories can be used to discover the root cause of your issue and begin the crucial initial steps towards overcoming it. They include:

How Did Your Pain Begin?

Are you aware that when you go to the doctor, they'll often begin by asking you to explain to them what occurred? There's a valid reason behind this: it aids the doctor in determine the root cause of the problem to a handful of.

The question you must think about how did this occur? Was it result of an injury? If yes What kind of injury did it suffer? Was it an injury from impact such as a twist or sprain? Did it happen slowly over a long duration?

The Specific Symptoms

Knee pain could be associated with various symptoms and conditions that aid in determining the cause of the issue.

Think about your personal symptoms. For instance, do you carry weight on that leg? Are you experiencing pain? If yes, are you suffering from pain all the time, regardless of effort or when you rest? Does your joint become locked? Does it appear like it's been bruised or deformed? Are you sure it's hot? Do you hear a popping or grinding sound while using it? Does it appear to be swelling? Do you experience a sensation of feeling full?

Where's Your In Pain?

The site of pain can help identify specific issues over other. Sometimes, pain is general rather than localized, however, it usually is some of the categories below:

It is the front of your knee (anterior knee pain) The front knee is the most frequently occurring area and is often due to muscle weakness, overuse , or small malalignment of the patella.

The knee's inner side It is often caused by cartilage and ligament tears or arthritis.

Behind knee: Most often due to arthritis, but sometimes a cartilage tear.

Outer side Outer side: This is the most frequent place. It could indicate ligament injury.

Below the knee Below the knee: Patellar Tendonitis (Jumpers Knie) or Osgood Schlatter's disease.

Keep in mind that these are general signs of the issue that you may suffer from. There is no substitute for a definitive diagnosis by a physician and therefore, ensure that you seek medical attention.

Chapter 3: Go To Your Doctor Right Away If...

It's difficult to tell if an condition or injury warrants urgent visits to A&E or a relaxing visit to the doctor at home or a few TLC remedies at home, such as rest and ice. You don't want to waste time or time and certainly don't want to finish appearing foolish. However, many knee injuries aren't able to wait and could cause permanent damage and pain if not dealt with quickly.

Get medical advice right away when you exhibit the following signs:

* You aren't able to put pressure on your knee in any way.

If you experience extreme discomfort even when you're lifting your knee, like in the evening.

* Your knee may lock or clicks painfully.

* Your knee opens under your feet.

* You're not able to fully bend or straighten your knee.

* Your knee looks deformed.

* You may experience an infection, redness or heat around the knee.

• Your knee has become very swelling.

* You are suffering from sensations of tingling or numbness in your leg below the knee area that you are affected by.

* The pain doesn't begin to get better within a few weeks, or you're experiencing discomfort that isn't gone after a couple of days of taking care of it at home.

You may cause yourself more issues by trying to ignore the pain and continue with your day, so ensure that you get evaluated.

Chapter 4: Most Significant Myths Regarding Knee Pain

A majority of us have knee pain at one moment in our lives. So when we are looking for relief, we look to the sources that we have a good idea of such as the internet, friends and families as well as the doctor or anyone else who would like to chip into the conversation with a few tips.

The issue is that everyone has their own methods and tricks that they claim to be the only way to treat your knee pain that's debilitating but you're left lost and often depressed before you've even started. The same goes for doctors. betterthan the average person. They often have their own motivations as well as their own goals and financial motives, and often choose to use painful injections or surgeries before they've truly grasped the problem.

How do you determine who you can trust? Are you confident that you'll feel relief and be capable of getting back to your feet and enjoy a normal lifestyle and not stumbling around like an old man?

Unfortunately, there are numerous myths surrounding knee pain and its solutions that can be frustrating, ineffective and painful when used improperly. This is why I thought it was important to write his book to help you make sure you're straight.

There is more power to treat your knees and ease the pain than you thought possible, and there's always possibility of recovery, even if you are unable to get up out of your chair. It's about recognizing the myths that exist as well as taking the health of your own hands to address the issue directly.

So , without further delay this is some of the most common myths surrounding the knee and its healing as well as some advice about what to do.

Myth #1 Cartilage can't heal

If you're confronted with a cartilage issue, it is common for your physician to recommend surgery, insisting that cartilage can't heal, and there's no other choice. This is a sham. While it is the case that cartilage recovers less quickly than other tissues within our bodies, the cartilage can healand, when it's given the proper care and the right environment, it'll heal without needing to use painful treatments.

Myth #2: Kne replacements and surgery are the only way to solve the problem.

Your knee hurts like hell and you've tried a variety of other treatments that don't even a smidgen of improvement. In desperation, you choose to undergo those costly and painful surgeries that transform your life, and sometimes not for the better.

There are many alternative options and various treatments that can assist in the resolution of the majority of your issues and heal your knees if you focus the issue directly, employing the tried and tested treatments we'll explore in the coming days.

Myth #3 You should never use ice for knee pain

It's generally recommended to apply ice to the knee pain or injury. It helps lessen swelling, reduce discomfort and reduce any discomfort you feel. I recommend that my patients apply the ice method in order to manage their individual issues. Although it's extremely helpful during the beginning stages it also constricts blood vessels within your knee, which can prolong the time needed to recover. Heating, contrary, increases blood flow and speeds up the healing process.

The most effective solution is to alternate both. If you've just been injured and causes discomfort, consider the recommended ice treatment in the treatment. After a trauma, think about alternating between the two.

Myth #4 If you're suffering from pain, you are damaged or broken.

If I had a dime for each time patients came to my office, trembling that they'd smashed or damaged anything, I'd extremely wealthy person indeed. There's an untruth that says that when you feel your knee hurts it means you've broken the bone or ruptured the tendon. This is a myth! A knee joint is complicated joint that is susceptible to all types of injury as well as the more severe kinds of injuries. The statistics show that you are much more likely to sustain an injury like a sprain or Patellofemoral Pain Syndrome than something less serious.

Do not be worried, get an official diagnosis from your physician instead.

Myth #5 that rest for the long-term is the only way to solve the problem

Say you're suffering from knee pain and you'll probably receive a frown from the person you're with and a clear advice to avoid using the limb in any way.

"Rest and rest, relax, relax!" is the mantra.

But with regards to the body's health, it certainly can be doing too much of an excellent thing. While rest is an excellent method to relieve the stress on joints and let it heal properly however, it can be extremely harmful if you stop training or activities completely. Your joints could actually'seize up' because of the lack of exercise, and the muscles weaken, and overall health will decrease as a result.

To ensure optimal healing, it is essential that you mix regular intervals of relaxation with moderate movement and exercises to ensure circulation to your affected area. Keep your muscles in good shape and ensure your body is healthy. Talk to your doctor or physiotherapist to get more details about how you can do this in a safe manner.

Chapter 5: Beware Of These Things If You Sustain An Injury

If you've hurt your knee no matter if it's from an accident, injury from sports or as a result of a different condition it is important to ensure that you're doing the right thing to avoid further damage and assist your knee heal as soon as is possible.

The majority of the advice is focused on what you ought to do, such as placing ice on your injured limb, or taking painkillers, but fails to discuss the things you must avoid. This section is devoted to the very same issues.

HARM

There's an acronym that refers to things to avoid in the period of 24 to 72 hours following any injury, or onset of knee pain. I'm sure you'll agree with me that they're very appropriate. This acronym stands for H.A.R.M.

What does it mean:

H stands for heat. Avoid using to any heat at this point because it can cause blood flow and swelling.

A is for alcohol. Do not drink alcohol within the first few days following the injury. It could delay healing.

R is for running. Absolutely no running or exercising following an injury. There is nothing at all.

M is a contraction of massage. Avoid massage on the region since it will increase swelling and causes bleeding.

Implement 'H.A.R.M to be on the right track to fast and efficient healing.

Chapter 6: The Long-Term Strategies That Work

Alongside the tips and advice in the sections specifically devoted to each condition and the treatment for it There are alternatives that can be implemented to preserve the strength and health of your knees and lessen the pain that you feel in the near future.

They're very easy to implement and won't require drastic changes in your life. Here's a list of them.

1. Always warm up and cool down prior to and after exercising.

2. Begin to gradually increase your level of exercise , but do not push yourself over your limit.

3. Be active and mobile, and ensure you do regular exercise on a daily schedule.

4. A healthy diet is essential to boost your health.

5. Build the muscles of your knee to assist in supporting the joint. Talk to your physiotherapist about the exact exercises you could perform.

Chapter 7: Knee Ailments Explained

In the next chapter, I will discuss every injury or condition which can cause knee pain in depth, including the causes as well as the symptoms and treatment options for each.

Now, go to the right section to your specific pain or go through them all to aid you determine the cause of your pain.

They include:

* Patellofemoral Pain Anterior Knee Pain/Syndrome

* Strains and Sprains

* Rheumatoid Arthritis

* Torn Hamstring

* Menisci Damage

* Chondromalacia Patella (Runner's Knee)

* Osteoarthritis

* Patellar Tendinitis (Jumper's Knee)

* Bursitis (Housemaid's knee)

Haemarthrosis (Bleeding through the Joint)

* Osgood-Schlatter's disease

* Gout

Patellofemoral Pain Syndrome/ Anterior Knee Pain

What exactly is it?

Patellofemoral discomfort is among the most prevalent kinds of knee pain there, and is the only one that's as mysterious. This makes it quite difficult to manage. It's because it often appears to be no evidence of any injury or damage to the knee it self.
What are the signs?

The signs and symptoms that are a sign of Patellofemoral Pain Syndrome include a grinding sound within your knee joint, faint sensation of fullness, pain that fades and comes back, and a mild swelling in the area. It may also be made worse when you use your knees in an unusual way like kneeling, squatting, or sitting for prolonged durations, walking uphill, or climbing stairs.

What are the causes?

Doctors believe that the reason is typically an increase in pressure between the femur and patella due to the overuse of exercise, excessive training, issues in the hips, or knee muscles or even a slight disalignment in the patella.

What can you do to treat it?

The standard treatment options of rest, painkillers , and the use of an ice-pack work well for this type of knee discomfort. Be sure to visit your doctor for an official diagnosis to rule out other serious knee issues.

An extremely effective method of treatment is also strengthening the muscles surrounding the knee by performing exercises that are not weight bearing, such as cycling, swimming and yoga.

It is also worth to seek the advice of a physiotherapist when other approaches don't assist. They may be able to perform a "taping of the kneecap' that is exactly as it sounds - the professional will apply tape externally to hold your kneecap and let the remaining knee to relax. Furthermore, they'll be able suggest specific exercises that can help you tackle the issue at home.

Strains and strains

What exactly is it?

A sprain can be described as a stretch or minor tearing of your ligaments . A strain is a stretch or tearing of tendon or muscle. Tendons are the tissues that connects bones to muscles. No matter what condition you're experiencing, they can create a great deal of discomfort and pain and may keep you off for several weeks.

What are the signs?

The symptoms include tenderness or pain and a distinct "pop" sound when you feel an injury. It can also be accompanied by swelling, possible bruising. You may also notice knees that flex when you try to load weight onto the knees.

What is the cause?

The most common cause of strains and sprains is doing more exercise or activity than you're accustomed to, and especially in the event that you did not stretch out to warm your muscles prior to exercising. It could result from sudden twists or related injuries.

What can you do to treat it?

The most effective method for treating any strain or strain is called PRICE therapy and painkillers. This can help reduce the pain, reduce swelling as well as internal bleeding and shorten the time to recover. What you should do:

Protection. (Optional depending on severity) Utilize a brace to secure your joint.

Rest. Don't engage in the sport that caused the injury. Rest the joint affected as long as is possible. Think about using crutches when walking.

Ice. Apply an Ice pack. Apply an ice pack (or even a packet of frozen vegetables) wrapped in towels for 20-minute intervals during the entire day. Don't apply ice directly to the skin because it could cause burns.

Compression. Apply a compression bandage on your body to stop bleeding and swelling.

Elevation. Lift your limb above your heart while you are asleep or resting to decrease swelling and encourage healing.

Painkillers

Choose a painkiller to ease your pain while you're suffering. I would highly recommend ibuprofen due to the anti-inflammatory properties it claims to have.

Lifestyle

Be sure to set aside enough time prior to engaging in any exercise to warm your muscles. Then, continue the process of cooling down' following. Do not just jump into intense levels of activity if your body has been lacking in activity for a long time. Instead, slow down and gradually increase the degree as your body gets more well-conditioned.

Think about your shoes you're wearing, for both work out and for use in everyday life. Make sure you are wearing low-heeled footwear like stilettos because they are often a cause of injuries to your ankles and knees, and you should invest in premium sports shoes that can provide shock absorption and safeguard your knees.

Rheumatoid Arthritis

What exactly is it?

Rheumatoid arthritis is an extremely serious autoimmune condition that affects the whole body, mainly the joints. The body has been triggered by something to defend itself, and the tissues it has in contrast to the tissues of foreign invaders like viruses and bacteria. This results in painful and swelling joints. It could occur at any point in time and not only as a result of ageing.

What are the signs?

The signs of rheumatoid arthritis typically include red and painful joints. They also experience swelling and warm around the knee, and general fatigue. There will be pain on both knees, and the pain is persistent and last for over an entire week. The joints of your knees are likely to be stiff when you get up in the morning, but they will also persist for the majority during the entire day. To top all of the above, you knee might be able to 'lock'.

What are the causes?

However, doctors aren't certain what triggers rheumatoid arthritis.

What can you do to treat it?

There isn't any effective treatment for rheumatoid joint and many doctors suggest pain relief, treatments to ease inflammation, and surgery to repair the damage that has occurred. But, many sufferers have found that making changes to their lifestyles aids, particularly those that address stress. This could include following an anti-inflammatory diet, or taking a look at the paleo diet and taking supplements with fish oil as well as going vegan or vegetarian as well as practicing the practice of yoga and meditation.

Torn Hamstring

What exactly is it?

A pulled or stretched Hamstring tends to be a frequent reason for knee pain in everyone of any age particularly athletes and people who lead very active lives.

The muscles of the hamstring are a collection of muscles that runs down in the back of the thighs. They enable users to stretch their legs. Although we often refer to it as a single muscle however, it's actually a collection comprised of 4 muscles. If you overuse the muscles it may stress or tear the muscle.

The hamstring is a muscle that runs from the hip to the end of the knee. So should the injury occur within the knee joint there will be discomfort there.

What are the signs?

If you've injured your hamstring, then you'll probably be aware of it quickly. You may notice a snapping sound or an erupting sensation after the injury took place. The pain may increase gradually or appear suddenly depending on the extent of the injury. It's possible that you'll be swollen and pain that radiates to the calf or thigh muscles and stiffness that develops after resting your knee.

How do you deal with it?

In the case of hamstring injuries It is recommended to follow the PRICE protocol as well as take anti-inflammatory painkillers like Ibuprofen. This can help reduce inflammation, decrease swelling, and internal bleeding , and speed up the time to recover. This is a quick reminder of what's involved:

Protection. (Optional depending on the severity) Utilize a brace to secure your joint.

Rest. Do not engage in the activities that led to the injury. Rest the joint affected as long as you can. Try using crutches for walking.

Ice. Apply an Ice pack. Apply the ice (or even a packet of frozen vegetables) wrapped in an absorbent towel for 20 minute intervals during the entire day. Don't apply ice directly to the skin since it can cause burns.

Compression. Use a compression bandage stop any further swelling and loss of blood.

Elevation. You can raise your limbs higher than your heart when you're asleep or resting to decrease swelling and encourage healing.

Lifestyle

Do not forget to warm up prior to exercise and cool down afterward to avoid further injuries in the future.

Menisci Damage

What exactly is it?

Menisci are tissues with pads located in your knee, in between the lower and upper leg bones. They serve as shock absorbers, and also protect the bones from collisions. Sometimes, they can tear or even twisted into the space around the joint, causing pain and issues.

What are the signs?

If the knee pain you are experiencing stems from menisci injuries, you'll suffer from intense pain, locking of the joint, and swelling in your joint. It is painful to carry any weight and may also hurt more when you attempt to move your knee.

What is the cause?

Menisci injuries are typically the final component of a serious injury like twisting or strike on the knee.

What are the best ways to deal with it?

In addition, the PRICE treatment plan is best for the immediate treatment of this type of knee issue and also for using anti-inflammatory painkillers like Ibuprofen. This will help to lessen the pain, reduce swelling as well as internal bleeding and shorten the time to recover. Here's a brief overview of the process:

Protection. (Optional depending on the severity) Use a brace secure your joint.

Rest. Don't engage in the activities that led to the injury. Rest the joint as long as you can. Think about using crutches when walking.

Ice. Apply an Ice pack. Make use of the ice (or even a packet of frozen vegetables) wrapped in towels for 20-minute intervals during the entire day. Do not apply ice directly on the skin because it could cause burns.

Compression. Use a compression bandage keep from bleeding and swelling.

Elevation. You can raise your limbs higher than your heart when you're asleep or resting to decrease swelling and speed up healing.

The treatment plan you choose to follow at this point will be a result of a range of variables like your age, the severity of your injury is, as well as the extent to which your injuries have impacted your life.

It's also a good idea to consider physiotherapy to help your joint move to promote healing, and avoid scar tissue growing, which could cause different joint problems later on. It is possible that you will require keyhole surgery in order to repair the injury, but it's typically not an option.

It is vitally important to consult your doctor as quickly as you can If you think you're suffering from damage to your menisciand if it is not treated, it can increase your chance of developing osteoarthritis later on.

Chondromalacia Patella (Runner's knee)

What exactly is it?

Chondromalacia patella can also be referred to as 'Runner's Knee' and is a condition that affects the cartilage of your knee. Cartilage is the connective tissue that runs along the edges of your bones. It allows them slide smoothly across each other without causing any injury. It also helps support the joint during motion, and acts as a powerful shock absorber for knees. If it is damaged or is not functioning properly it can cause pain and decreases the range of motion.

What are the signs?

The signs and symptoms of Chondromalacia Patella consist of a mild painful ache at the knee's front swelling, as well as an increase in pain working with the joint, particularly when bent knees while walking up a flight of steps or kneeling for long time. There is a decrease in range of motion as well as the sensation of tightness and feeling of fullness.

What are the causes?

The reasons for this aren't completely clear however it's probable that it's due to injuries or overuse, arthritis, or an infection.

What are the best ways to deal with it?

It is believed that cartilage does not contain its own source of oxygen, and consequently, these types of knee injuries can be difficult to heal. The standard treatment is to use nonprescription painkillers as well as anti-inflammatory drugs like Ibuprofen as well as non-steroidal anti-inflammatory medications called NSAIDs. Additionally the patient is often advised to undergo physiotherapy in order to stimulate the knee to heal or surgery to stimulate the growth of cartilage, or even a complete knee replacement.

But, in my personal experience, it is too invasive and could be risky. Every procedure comes with the risk of complications and it's always better to prompt your body's healing process and enhance the overall health of joints. The trick is to slowly increase the amount of activity in your joint, and to use exercises that are not weight-bearing, such as cycling or swimming to boost the flow of blood, build up surrounding muscles and encourage healing. It's true that this may take longer than the majority of tissues however, a dose of patience can help in helping your body heal naturally.

It is important to visit your doctor if think you suffer with Chondromalacia Patella to determine if there are any other grave issues. However, make sure that you don't take any treatment plans and instead seek another opinion.

Osteoarthritis

What exactly is it?

Osteoarthritis is among the most prevalent causes of knee pain particularly as we age. But, you don't need to be old to suffer from it. A lot of older people are also affected by osteoarthritis due to an injury, and especially in the event that the injury goes untreated. It's the wear-and tear form of arthritis, which happens when cartilage becomes damaged and bone surfaces are unprotected and prone to damage and friction. As you'd expect , it's mostly in hips and knees.

What are the signs?

If you suffer with osteoarthritis, then you'll be experiencing swelling in the knee and related issues. You may experience stiffness when you awake in the morning. This improves after one hour or so. Your pain will ease as you take a break from your joints, but you may feel more so after you've used them. Sometimes, your knees could become stiff or painful.

What are the causes?

The majority of cases of osteoarthritis are due to an injury or normal wear and tear of a joint during the course of a lifetime. It is also possible to have the result of a genetic predisposition which can manifest earlier in the course of.

Obesity is also a contributing factor to osteoarthritis because of the increased weight that is placed on the knees and the risk of infections. Previous untreated injuries can also increase the chance of being affected by this kind of knee issue.

What can you do to treat it?

If you suspect that you're suffering from osteoarthritis, it's vital that you consult your physician to seek additional advice and to rule out any other issues.

There isn't a cure for osteoarthritis, however there are many options to treat the symptoms you are experiencing using conventional as well as alternative therapies so that you can receive the most effective type of relief you can get.

Ibuprofen, a painkiller, is a great option for osteoarthritisbecause of their anti-inflammatory properties. Also, consider physical therapy that can help build up the muscles surrounding the knee region and help diagnose any postural issues that may cause pain.

The proper type of footwear will have a huge impact on your symptoms, as will the elimination of any excess weight that you may have.

You could also think about supplementing with fish oils or Glycosamine Sulphate. Through studies, both these products have produced positive results in treating arthritis and other types of bone and muscle problems.

Additionally, a lot of people are adamant about "Tiger Balm". It's an Chinese massage balm that comes in a small container and is said to perform wonders for all kinds of muscular or joint discomfort. I'm yet to test this for myself, but If my experience with patients is any indication I'd strongly suggest that you try it.

Joint replacement could be a possibility when you're experiencing a drastic decrease in your quality of life due to being afflicted by osteoarthritis. But, it's not something that should be taken lightly, so make sure you consult a specialist and consider all alternatives first.

Patellar Tendinitis (Jumper's Knee)

What exactly is it?

Tendonitis refers to an swelling of the tendon which is the elastic band of tissue that connects the muscle with the bone. It is commonly referred to as 'Jumper's Knee' because it is a common affliction for players of sports like netball, basketball, in trampolining or other sports that require running or jumping. The inflammation causes movements that is painful as well as restricted.

What are the signs?

In addition to pain and limited mobility You may also suffer from discomfort, swelling, and redness. The pain will likely be more severe when you place pressure on your knee, go between the stairs, or even attempt at walking faster than normal. The pain will likely occur below the kneecap, at the point where the tibia bone begins.

What are the causes?

The constant jumping during sports puts strain on the tendons. This can result in them becoming painful, leading to the pain you're feeling.

How do you deal with it?

Tendonitis is often portrayed as less severe than it is and the discomfort and pain that it causes could last weeks sometimes even up to months. The most effective method of approach is to adopt the PRICE treatment plan that helps accelerate recovery, lessen discomfort and assist in getting the swelling to a minimum. It comprises:

Protection. (Optional depending on the severity) Use a brace ensure your joint is protected.

Rest. Do not engage in the sport that caused the injury. Rest the joint affected as long as is possible. Try using crutches for walking.

Ice. Apply an Ice pack. Apply an ice pack (or even a packet of frozen vegetables) wrapped in an absorbent towel for 20 minute intervals during the entire day. Do not apply ice directly on the skin because it could cause burns.

Compression. Use a compression bandage stop any further swelling and loss of blood.

Elevation. Lift your limb above your heart while you are sleeping or resting to minimize swelling and speed up healing.

Furthermore be sure to take adequate painkillers that ease the discomfort. It is recommended to use ibuprofen whenever possible since it has anti-inflammatory properties that can be particularly useful in treating tendonitis. Visit your physician to get advice on other painkillers or methods of treatment you can try.

It could also include physiotherapy sessions to strengthen and stretch the injured tendons as well as surrounding muscles, in addition to identifying your daily movements that could be contributing to the issue.

Many take corticosteroids shots around the injured tendon, which may help reduce pain and inflammation. It is usually administered along with an anesthetic local to the area that decreases the pain. The procedure itself is extremely painful (speaking from personal experience) however it can also provide substantial benefits when your life is seriously affected by tendonitis. Be sure to allow at minimum one month between sessions, and do not exceed three injections at the injured location.

Surgery is usually utilized as the last option for issues that aren't getting resolved after several months. It is performed through the removal of the injured part of the tendon and removing the deposits that have been formed, and repairing the damage or promoting healing, typically through keyhole surgery. However, it could cause negative side effects, and should be avoided in the extent that is feasible.

Bursitis (Housemaid's knee)

What exactly is it?

The cause of bursitis is inflammation of small bursa, a sack filled with liquid that are located in the places in which the tendons and ligaments cross bones, for instance on the knee. If they are subjected to excessive amounts of friction, for instance, kneeling, they can become painful, and inflamed. In addition, the volume of fluid inside the sacks increases and makes movement difficult.

What are the signs?

The signs of bursitis are hot, tender and red joints, as well as apparent swelling. The pain gets worse when you bend or kneel your knee. It is often felt like an unrelenting ache. There is also a restricted mobility within the joint.

If the pain persists and the redness gets worse or you experience fever, you should consult your physician as soon as possible. You might suffer from septic bulsitis and require prompt treatment.

What are the causes?

It's also known as "Housemaid's Knee" because it's usually caused by kneeling for prolonged periods of time, which is what housekeepers would do in past times. Today, it's typically plumbers, carpet-layers, or other individuals who suffer the most. The most painful and risky type, Septic Bursitis, is caused by an infection of the bursa.

How do you deal with it?

The most effective treatment for bursitis is to rest. It's essential that you refrain from moving your knees while you are recuperating of the irritation. It is also possible to use the ice pack for 20 minutes all day long to decrease the swelling and pain. It's also helpful to lift your knee over your heart as high as is possible and especially while at rest or sitting. It is important to be sure to avoid sleeping on this side to safeguard your knee from injury , and to also help lessen swelling.

Painkillers like aspirin Paracetamol, and Ibuprofen are also extremely effective, as are the non-steroidal anti-inflammatory medications (NSAIDs). If you suffer from Septic Bursitis then you'll have to undergo a regimen of antibiotics that are strong to fight the disease. Please consult your physician for an expert diagnoses as well as treatment alternatives.

If the inflammation does not heal on its own, you may look into treatment with either surgery or aspiration. The surgeon or doctor will be able to remove the excessive fluid from your knee with scalpel or a needle. The best option is to cut off the affected bursa, but that isn't the only option.

Another option is to get corticosteroid injections to the area affected. It is important to leave an interval of at least six weeks between injections, and make sure you do not have over three shots to the affected area in order to avoid adverse consequences.

It is highly recommended that you also start using knee pads that are protective in the near future to prevent the possibility of recurrence.

Haemarthrosis (Bleeding to the Joint)

What exactly is it?

If you've injured an ligament, fractured bones or suffer from hemophilia, you may suffer from joint bleeding that causes swelling and discomfort. The medical term for it is Haemarthrosis and may cause lasting injury.

What are the signs?

Haemarthrosis makes it nearly impossible for your knee to be moved and it'll be warm and stiff, as well as swelling. It is possible to experience external bruising and feeling a bubbling , or discomfort within the joint. The joint will expand significantly due to.

What are the causes?

Hemophilia and injury are the main causes of joint bleeding. However, it could be experienced by anyone, and especially those who are taking blood thinners.

What can you do to treat it?

It is essential to get medical attention right away If you think you're experiencing bleeding from your knee because you must stop the bleeding in order to repairs are needed and to prevent the development of arthritis due to.

This is especially true in cases of severe swelling.

Like all knee issues, it's essential to rest the knee as well as apply ice to decrease swelling, and use painkillers like ibuprofen when is needed.

Be sure to do regular exercises to strengthen the muscles that surround your knees. This will aid in preventing future issues.

Osgood-Schlatter's disease

What exactly is it?

The one with the fancy name and , while it can cause a amount of pain but it's not as severe as it may sound. It's a common occurrence among kids who are extremely active and engage in a variety of sports, particularly ones that require running and jumping. It's also connected to the growth spurts which occur at puberty.

What are the signs?

The discomfort can range from chronic and debilitating to mild and intermittent dependent on what's causing the issue. It's typically experienced on one knee, however it could also manifest in both. It is possible to find an unidentified bony lump beneath the knee. If the joint is swelling and red, or becomes locked or unstable, or the child has fever, it's crucial to seek medical attention immediately.

What are the causes?

Repetitive activity causes the tendon that connects the kneecap and the leg below to shift off from the bone leading to pain and swelling. It could also cause a bony growth appear just above the top of the shin which can cause further discomfort.

What can you do to treat it?

It's difficult to convince children who are active to take a break and rest, but it's crucial to recovery. Also, make sure you take enough painkillers like Paracetamol or Ibuprofen and apply the ice (wrapped with a towels) for 20 minutes often throughout the day. The problem will go away in some weeks or even months, but it may recur until your child's growth has been completed.

Gout

What exactly is it?

Gout is a disease which is typically associated with those who are wealthy, however in reality, anyone is susceptible to its symptoms. It's actually a form of arthritis that triggers painful and swelling joints all over your body. It's not only in knee joints.

What are the signs?

If you suffer from gout, then you'll be prone to sudden bouts of intense knee pain. your knee will appear hot and red. It is common to feel pain while you rest and at night, and not just when you try to work the joint affected. It is possible to be suffering from gout in other areas of your body as well like the joints of your hands and feet.

What is the cause?

It's caused due to a build-up of crystallized uric acids inside the knee. Uric acid acts as a degrading material and can cause pain and inflammation. It's usually caused by overweight and purines-rich foods as well as drinking large amounts of alcohol, and taking certain medicines.

How do you deal with it?

Prior to that, treat the knee by applying ice packs for 20 minutes several at a time during the course of your daily life. using painkillers like Paracetamol and Ibuprofen as well as taking non-steroidal anti-inflammatory medications (NSAIDs).

It's also crucial to keep your limb from being knocked down at issue and elevate your limb when you're at rest or sitting.

Diet plays a significant role with the development of gout so it is essential that you alter your diet to stay away from food items that are rich in purines, which can raise the levels of uric acids in your body , which can trigger problems. This includes avoiding offal, game oils, seafood, and fish as well as food items that contain yeast extract or malt extract, as well as taking steps to reduce any excess weight.

Also, cut down on intake of alcohol and engage in more exercises to allow your body break down the Uric acid instead of storage.

Chapter 8: The Different Knee Problems, Conditions, And Injuries

Many knee injuries result from knee injuries. The sudden or acute injuries typically result from an unintentional blow to the knee or due to abrupt bending, irregular twisting or directly impacting the knee. If injuries of this kind occur typically, they result in swelling and bruising and discomfort. There could also be weakness and numbness as well as swelling and bruising can occur within minutes, since certain nerves or blood vessels may be damaged in the course of the injury. The most frequent knee injuries could comprise:

* Strains and strains as well as other injuries related to the ligaments, tendons and muscles that connect and support the kneecap.

A tear is forming in the elastic and tough cushioning within the joint of knee.

* Tearing the anteriorcruciate ligament or medial collateral ligament which is the most often injured ligament.

* Injuring the kneecap, which is damaged when it is struck by a powerful force like hitting your kneecap, twisting it violently and then bending it in a way that is abnormally.

* Relocating the kneecap.

* Loss of bones or tissues that are caused by fractures or dislocations that are trapped in the joint, restrain knee movement.

* The knee joint is dislocated. A dislocated knee joint can be an extremely serious injury and should be addressed immediately.

Apart from acute or sudden injury, there's injuries from overuse that happen due to repetitive activities or extended tension to the knee. The repetitive activities can comprise walking, climbing stairs cycling and running, jumping and so on. The most frequent injuries sustained from overuse be:

* Inflammation or bursitis of small sacs filled with liquid that cushion and lubricate knee joints. This is often a result of an injury that results from injuries or overuse.

The cause is inflammation in the tendon or tear of the tendon.

* The stiffening or folding of the knee ligaments called the plica syndrome.

* Knee pain in front due to knee injuries, excessive use excessive weight or issues within the kneecap.

* Irritation or inflammation on the fibrous tissue which runs along the outside of the thigh.

* Inflammation of the cartilage beneath the kneecap, causing knee discomfort. This type of inflammation typically is seen in younger people.

* Knee osteoarthritis. It is an arthritis type that is extremely common in elderly people. This is often caused by age and regular wear and tear on cartilage. Signs of knee osteoarthritis include swelling, pain and stiffness.

* Knee effusion. It is the process by which fluid accumulates inside the knee as a result of swelling caused by an injury.

* Injuring the meniscus which comprises the cartilage which cushions and helps protect the knee. The injury usually occurs after the knee has been badly bent. Meniscus damage that is severe result in massive tears that result in the knee locking.

* A tear in the anterior cruciate ligament can cause the knee's instabilityand causes it to rupture suddenly. This type of tear might require surgical repair.

* Straining or tears the ligament of the posterior cruciate. This can result in pain, swelling and instability. These injuries occur less frequently than ACL and are able to be treated by undergoing physical therapy.

The tear or strain of the collateral ligament medial can cause discomfort and instability to the inside of the knee.

* Patellar subluxation--abnormality of the kneecap which slides or dislocates along the thigh bone during certain activities.

* Patellar tendonitis. This is the irritation or inflammation of the tendon connecting the kneecap and shin bone. This type of injury typically affects athletes.

* The accumulation of fluid at the back of the knee , referred to as"baker's Cyst. This kind of injury usually occurs as due to arthritis.

It is prevalent in older people, may cause arthritis in any joint of the body. This condition needs to be addressed immediately, since when left untreated, it can cause irreparable damage to the joints.

* Gout is also a typical form of arthritis caused by the build-up of uric acids or crystals in joints, including the knee.

* Pseudogout is an additional type of arthritis that is like gout. However, it's caused by the accumulation in calcium pyrophosphate crystals inside the knee joint as well as in other joints.

It is caused due to bacteria in the knee. It can result in swelling, pain, inflammation and difficulty in walking with the knee. While this kind of arthritis is not as common but it is still important to get it immediately treated since it is likely to worsen if it is not treated.

What should you be aware of about knee pain

There is wear and tear that occurs on our knee joints along with the inevitable joint pains and aches that go from it, are a typical aspect of ageing. The most frequently reported joint issues is knee pain.

Many people prefer to ignore knee pain. However it is a good idea to keep complaining about the pain in your knees and if your discomfort persists for longer than a week or two It is recommended to rest and consult your doctor to get an assessment. The intensity or frequency of pain in the knee differs from person to. Knee pain is more frequent when you play many sports, and also among older individuals. The majority of the time, knee pain can appear on the either the front or back of your knee. The cause of the pain is usually caused by an imbalance in the muscles that affects the kneecap's ability to take on the strains during movement.

Athletes are more likely to suffering knee pain or other injuries as a result of their strenuous exercises. However, the overuse of knees is one of the most common causes of knee discomfort. Knee pain can treat at-home. By resting, applying cold or hot compresses, along with elevation will get rid of discomfort. If the persistent pain persists, it's important to see a doctor to be examined for knee pain and assessed.

How to prevent and treat knee discomfort on your own

Tips to help prevent knee pain with natural methods

Maintain your weight in a healthy way. To ensure that your knees are solid and fit, it's essential to maintain an appropriate weight. Each pound you put on adds around 4 pounds of strain on your knees each time you walk up and down stairs or walk. Patients suffering from knee pain that managed to shed some of their excess weight eventually will be free of the symptoms of knee pain and also the knee pain in itself.

Be careful not to climb either way or down steps. This is crucial unless you're in excellent fitness. If you're already suffering from pain or weakness in your knees, you should avoid getting up and down steps. When you are weighing 120lbs, that implies that you have about 480 pounds of strain going into your knees. If you have to walk through the steps, be sure you are firmly seated on the railing to support yourself.

* Walk on hard, flat surfaces. Make sure to walk on concrete pathways or other surfaces so long as they're smooth and sturdy. Avoid walking on cobblestones and grass as their unevenness could create more stress and strain on your knees, and increase the likelihood of getting tripped up.

Be careful not to overdo your exercise routines. If you are doing exercises which require you to extend your knees to the side, be sure you don't do it more than 90 degrees.

• Work out your inner thighs. If your inner thigh muscles remain strong, they are more able to absorb the strain that comes with walking. This prevents knee strain.

* Adjust exercise bikes. Be careful not to sit in a position that is too low for your workout bikes. Adjust your seat and ensure that it's sufficiently high that your knee is able to straighten as the pedal falls to its lowest.

• Wear comfortable shoes. Be sure to have shoes that provide adequate cushioning for your feet and are sized to fit your foot. Shoes that are comfortable can help you maintain proper posture and stability in order to keep you from tripping and suffering knee injuries.

"Wake up. Don't forget to warm-up before you begin any type of exercise. Stretching your muscles prior to any type of activity can reduce the tension in your tendons. This relieves the stress on your knees.

* Choose to do low-impact exercises. Select exercises that place less stress on your knees such as using a rowing machine , or an equipment for cross country skiing.

* Swim or walk. Take a walk and swim to build your muscles, while not putting excessive stress onto your knees.

• Do some weight-training. It is crucial to build the muscles in your legs to not put too much stress onto your knees. Make sure you consult with a professional trainer before you start so that he or will be able to teach you how to properly weight train to avoid knee discomfort.

* Don't cut down on your activities. Many people avoid or limit their exercises to prevent knee discomfort. But it's advised not to limit your activities, since doing so could result in weakness, which may increase the chance of injury to your knee.

* Do not increase in intensity during your exercise. While you might want to build your knees and legs it is not advisable to abruptly alter your routine. Be sure to raise the intensity slowly, so that your knees and legs can adapt and adapt to the demands.

Do not lift large objects. Avoid attempting to lift objects that weigh a lot even if you're struggling to do it, since the pressure placed on your knee could cause it to fall and then break.

Avoid standing on unstable objects. Avoid standing on chairs that are unstable since there is an increased chance that you'll slip and fall onto your knees.

Wear knee protectors. Be sure to wear knee protectors that are safe for you during your sport or other activities for recreation.

Select the correct equipment. Do not use equipment that is greater than your capacity, size and strength.

• Avoid wearing high-heeled footwear. High heels can cause a lot of stress to your knees. Therefore, ensure that you aren't wearing heels that are high.

Eat nutritious foods. Foods that contain nutrients for your requirements. This includes yogurt, milk and dark greens leafy vegetables, cheese and other leafy greens.

* Reduce your consumption of alcohol. Avoid drinking excessive amounts of alcohol drinks. If you're a man limit yourself to two daily drinks of alcohol and for women you should limit yourself to one. Drinking alcohol can cause bone weakness and make them more susceptible to osteoporosis.

Stop smoking. For healthy bones It is crucial to quit smoking since smoking cigarettes, like alcohol, can make bones weaker, making them more susceptible to osteoporosis. Smoking also affects the flow of blood which flows across your feet, slowing down the process of healing.

How to treat knee discomfort naturally

You can try physical therapy. Physical therapy or occupational therapy can be highly beneficial for those suffering with knee discomfort. Therapists can design an exercise plan that is appropriate to your capabilities and needs. Apart from that they also will show you how to reduce the strain on your knees during your daily routine.

Relax and rest. Resting enough is just as crucial as working out or engaging in physical exercises. Relaxation and rest can to improve health, ease discomfort and allow your muscles time to recover.

* Make sure to get enough rest. Knee discomfort, and arthritis, could make getting an enjoyable night's rest impossible. But, it's important to sleep enough to allow your muscles to rest.

Make use of a hot or cold compress. If you are experiencing knee pain, you can ease it yourself by using a cold or hot compress to ease swelling and pain, or hot compresses to ease stiffness. Also, taking showering or bathing with hot water may help alleviate the pain.

Apply a topical pain relief. There are many available creams sprays, patches, sprays and gels available to ease knee pain. Even though they're not prescription-only however, it is important that you consult with your doctor to determine which one is suitable for you to utilize.

Drink an oral painkiller. Like topical pain reliefs there are several oral pain relievers that can help reduce knee pain. Before taking this medication but, ensure that you consult with your doctor first.

* Take a sip of turmeric and ginger tea. Drinking ginger and turmerictea, that are both naturally anti-inflammatory will help ease arthritis and knee pain. Turmeric has properties that to reduce the enzymes that cause knee inflammation. In order to make the tea you'll require 2 cups water 1 teaspoon crushed ginger 1 teaspoon of ground turmeric , and honey.

Bring the water to a boil then add the turmeric and ginger and then add honey.

* Soak your legs. Another way to ease knee pain is to soak the legs with warm water with Epsom salt. Epsom salt is a source of magnesium sulfate that has been proven to ease pain for a long time. To create this, all you need is 1 cup Epsom salt as well as warm water, and an enormous bowl.

* Increase your magnesium intake. All of us require magnesium, however, our bodies can't create it by themselves. Magnesium is a vital mineral, because it plays a role in relaxing muscles and nerves, as well as alleviating stiffness and pain. People who have diets that are rich in magnesium, or who took supplements are more bone-strong as well as higher density of bones.

* Take a drink of blackstrap Molasses. Blackstrap Molasses is a rich source of minerals, which include magnesium calcium, and potassium. It has been proven to alleviate various signs and discomforts that are that are associated with knee and arthritis paindue to the essential elements in it which regulate nerve and muscle functions as well as strengthen bones. To make this drink all you

require is 1 teaspoon of blackstrap-molasses as well as 1 cup of hot water.

Make an eucalyptus eucalyptus oil blend. The combination of eucalyptus with peppermint will help ease knee pain as a result of their healing properties. When they are applied to joints that are in pain or knees, the cooling effect can help relieve discomfort and pain which allows you to be relaxed. To create an oil blend, you'll require five drops of eucalyptus oil five drops peppermint oil 1 tablespoon carrier oil, and an unassuming glass bottle and, ideally, a dark bottle.

Rehab motivation

If you're experiencing knee pain, discomfort or you've injured yourself or are experiencing a tough getting around, your doctor could recommend physical therapists to assist you in restoring the strength of your knee and mobility, endurance, and mobility.
A lot of people are attracted to physical therapy. It's because they're amazed by the things they can accomplish when they are treated. But, physical therapy is an enormous amount of work and anyone who has to undergo physical therapy must anticipate that certain treatments and exercises may result in

some discomfort or pain. Some individuals are required to undergo a long-term course of physical rehabilitation. This leads them losing motivation. Due to the effort and the pain that comes with the therapy, it might appear like a huge burden to get up and go for the therapy.

There is a need for motivation while undergoing the process of physical rehabilitation. Motivation can be based on biological, cultural, or social factors that vary from person to person. For athletes who have injured their knees, they could be motivated to train hard to get back to playing their favorite sport as well as heart attack patients who undergo rehabilitation for their heart may be driven to continue their rehabilitation so that they can be released from the hospital and back to their lives as normal. Whatever the injury, rehabilitation motivation is vital to ensure that people can continue their rehabilitation and continue to get better.

To remain motivated during rehabilitation from physical therapy there are a few aspects you should take into consideration:

* Your physical Therapist. To ensure that you are involved in your rehabilitation program It is crucial that you choose the correct physical

therapy. Before you begin your treatment, don't be reluctant to ask the specialist specific questions to ensure that you're comfortable with the therapist and that they is the best fit for you. Your physical therapist must be able to inspire and inspire you, and also be someone you are able to get along with. If you are feeling that your physical therapist isn't capable of helping you don't hesitate to inquire about another person who is in a position to assist you with your physical rehab.

* Determine your progress. Physical therapists perform an assessment of your information and measurements prior to beginning your rehabilitation. It is possible to inquire from your physical therapist about to determine what the measurements you have taken and goals are. Your physical therapist will be able to assist you in progressively helping you reach your goals.

• Make friends with other patients. Being around people you trust can make your things much better. When you are in physical therapy, it is very likely that you will meet other patients similar to you and who are going through the same treatment as you. It is a good idea to try to start a conversations with fellow patients as having conversations with that there are others like you can inspire you to keep going with your rehabilitation.

You can listen to your own music. Music is a positive motivator as an appropriate music selection can influence individuals' moods. Talk to your physical therapist if it is possible to listen to your music while you receive treatment.

The process of recovering from an injury is very difficult. It's a long process that takes perseverance, determination and lots of time. At some point in your treatment, you could think that nothing is happening and your motivation might begin to wane. It is crucial not to dwell on these thoughts and instead concentrate on the things that can keep you motivated and assist to keep you on track with recovery. When you work with a therapist who's capable of encouraging and supporting you and hopefully, you'll be able to locate the appropriate amount of motivation to remain motivated, engaged and focused throughout the course of your rehabilitation.

Knee exercises to help with knee pain relief

If you're suffering from knee pain, you must realize that it's never too late to begin treating the knees as well as strengthening them. Even if you've suffered knee injuries or other issues, you can work out the muscles that surround the knee joints, such as the quadriceps muscles, hamstrings, the adductor and abductor, to make your knees more healthy and stronger. This will make them less susceptible to injuries. Regular exercise will prevent your joints from getting stiff and provides them with required support they require, allowing them to move with ease without discomfort that comes with it. To get you started, here are a few essential exercises are easy to do to strengthen your knees.

* Stretches

O Chair knee extension. Two chairs are needed and you can place one on the floor. Put your feet on the other chair, so you have your knee slightly raised. Gradually push your knee to the floor with only the muscles in your legs. Do this for 5-10 seconds before releasing. Repeat this for the other leg, and repeat the exercise 5 times.

A Heel-knee extension. Find a flat, comfortable floor and place your feet upon your back. Bend your left knee , and ensure that your left foot is level across the ground. Slowly move off your right heel until your legs are in line with each the other. Do this for 5-10 seconds before returning to your starting position. Repeat five times before repeating the process for the second leg.

Bend your knees. You can sit on a chair, and place a towel on your feet that is meant to lie in a flat position on the ground. Keep each end of your towel and gradually move them upwards to bend your knee until it's about 4 to 5 inches higher than the floor. You should hold it for five to 10 seconds, then let it go. Repeat 5 times, and then repeat the process for the second leg.

o Hamstring stretch. Standing up, place one toe in front, with your feet up. Set both hands onto the back of your back. Alternatively, you can hold the chair in place to help you stability. The knee should be bent in front of your body, as well as your hip until you feel your hamstrings are stretched. Do not reduce your lower back. Maintain the position for 5-10 seconds before releasing. Repeat the exercise five times, and then repeat exactly the same thing with the other leg.

* Strength training

A Wall slide. Get up and lean back against the wall. Bend your knees around 30 degrees, then slide across the wall and then up. Be sure to move slowlyand keep your palms on the wall to ensure security. To keep your equilibrium ensure that your feet and legs parallel and make sure not to allow your knees to extend beyond the toes. Repeat this exercise 5 or 10 times.

o Bent-leg raises. You can sit on a stool then straighten the left foot up. Keep it for 1 minute. Slowly bend your knee until it is it is about halfway down. Keep the position for 30 seconds and then return to the original position. Repeat this four times, and repeat the exercise with the opposite leg.

o Straight-leg raises. Sit in a chair, and put one foot on a different chair. Then, lift your foot just a few inches from the chair, but try that your leg remains straight. Keep this position for 5-10 seconds, then return to your resting position. Repeat the exercise 5-10 times, before repeating the exercise on the opposite leg. You can also gradually increase the duration and keep your leg in place for 2-3 minutes, if you are able to.

o Abductor raise. Find a flat and comfortable area and lay on your back and propped up on your elbow. Bend the leg that is on the floor , and maintain the other leg straight. Gradually lift the leg to the its top for 5-10 minutes before lowering it. If you are able then, you could also try using ankle weights. Perform 3 to 4 sets, with between 12 and 15 reps. Place your body on the opposite side and repeat the exercise with the opposite leg.

Hamstring curl. Place yourself on an area such as a table or wall to ensure your thighs are in the direction of an object. Lift one knee and bend it to the extent that is comfortable. Maintain this position for 5-10 seconds, then slowly lower it. Repeat the exercise 12-to-15 times being sure that you don't get your feet on the floor during repetitions. Perform 3 to 4 sets, then repeat the exercise with the second leg.

Step ups. Choose a chair or stairs and step up to it. Place your feet on the stairs or bench while straightening your knees then lower them. Repeat this exercise for one minute and gradually increase the time. Once you've found your balance You can also attempt to pump your arms while going between up and down.

o A stationary bicycle. A stationary bike can be a fantastic option for strengthening your knees. But, you must be sure to adjust the seat according to your height, so that your legs do not feel stressed. Begin by exercising on the bike for 10 minutes at a time and gradually increase the time.

Don't be too intense while exercising. Based on your abilities and existing level of movement, it's ideal to begin with stretching exercises, and then a little of strengthening exercises. You can then gradually increase the duration and level of your workout. Stretching should be practiced every day to avoid the joints from becoming stiff and stiffening.

Whatever exercises you do however, ensure you talk to your doctor whether these exercises are actually beneficial to you and won't cause you to risk becoming injured. If you feel pain during the exercise you should stop right away and consult an expert so that he or they can determine what's wrong.

Additionally, it's common to feel sore when you do certain exercises. If you experience this, apply ice to your knees for 10 - 20 mins. Take a cold compress or bag of frozen vegetables and cover it in the towel. Apply it to the joint and then raise your leg.

Chapter 9: Exercises For Strengthening

A strong, healthy muscle around the knee is strong pillars that prevent the cartilage of the articular region from coming into contact with one another. For OA knee, muscle strength exercises aid in restoring the normal biomechanics of knees, which results in a lower joint load rate or localized strain in the cartilage articular.

A strong muscle plays a significant role in preventing the onset and reducing the development of knee OA(Fransen and colleagues.).

Muscle strengthening is often referred to as muscle resistance exercises. Muscle strength is strengthened through resistance exercise (RX) improves physical performance and reduces pain from OA and decreases the self-reported impairment (Kevin R. Vincent, 2012).

Parts of a program for strengthening include

1. Resistance load

2. Repetitions,

3. The speed of movement as well as

4. The frequency of sessions each week.

An ongoing increase in resistance load during each exercise will allow for continual muscle adaptations in the course of time. Resistance can be applied using different techniques.

"Body weight": In this case it's the weight of the leg.

* Resistance bands, like Theraband.

* Free weights: We will be using a weight cuff.

* Machines.

All of the exercises we're going to talk about will follow an established routine of exercises three days a week. There will be three sets per exercise with 8-15 repetitions for each set.

Let's get our exercise routines going.

1. Static Quadriceps Exercises

Start position

Figure 8

Position of the target

Figure 9

The description of static quadricep exercises

The exercise is also known as knee press. It's called static since there's no joint movement when exercising, however there's plenty that muscles contract.

This type of exercise is crucial in cases of extremely severe knee pain. It is, however, the most vital exercise that is often prescribed by surgeons, doctors and physical therapists too.

The most appealing aspect of this exercise is that it fits in all the three phases of OA and is easy to master and practice. Before we can understand the importance of this exercise as well as the muscles it helps it, let's get acquainted with its method.
Technique

Figure 10

1. Lay on your back, flat as illustrated in the image.

2. A pillow (or sheets or towels) under the knee.

3. Press the pillow, and keep it in the position that you press for 5 minutes (count 5) before releasing it.

4. Repeat this exercise 30 minutes in one session, at least three times per day.

5. When pain is lessened, it can be repeated as many times as is comfortable.

The importance of quadricep exercises that are static

This exercise will help strengthen your quadriceps muscles. It is the most powerful muscle in our body, which is a set of four muscles located in side of the thighs. This is the reason it is called quadriceps i.e. quad= four, ceps=muscles. Take a look at the bulky muscles in the front of your thigh. They are the quadriceps muscles.

All four muscles are derived from the various regions of the ilium (front portion of hip bone) and join to form the quadriceps tendon. They connect to the upper portion of kneecap (patella bones).

The picture below illustrates the quadriceps muscle as well as its two segments which are the vastus latis and the rectus femoris.

Figure 11

It performs a vital role in extensing the knee joint which is why when this muscle is activated, it creates a an extension motion to the joint of knee.

For those suffering from symptomatic osteoarthritis in the knee area, quadriceps muscles weakening is commonplace and generally believed to be the result of an atrophy due to disuse that is caused by joint pain(Slemenda and colleagues.).

Bullet points

1. This workout helps to strengthen of the quadriceps muscles. Quadriceps muscles are located just in front of the thigh.

2. The role of the muscle is to expand the knee joint.

3. The most distinctive feature of this workout is that it's done with no motion or movement of joint. This is the reason it is known as "static".

***

2. Dynamic Quadriceps Exercises

Contrary to the previous quadriceps exercise, this workout requires movement of the limb and that is why it is referred to as a dynamic exercise. Another name for it is straight leg raise.

Start position

Figure 12

The target posture

Figure 13

Description of exercises for quadriceps that are dynamic and challenging.

This is also known as straight leg raise in which you have to raise the leg while keeping the your knee joint straight. Be aware that in contrast to the exercises mentioned above during this one, there is movement in the joint of your hip. This is the reason it is known as dynamic quadriceps exercises.

Note that it is the body's weight that acts as a resistance. When we are progressing through this exercise, it is possible to add weight, starting by adding half a kilogram weight in order to be more restraining. Then, we can continue to progress by adding 0.5 kg until we come the total of 2 kilograms of weight.

We recommend adding some weight with the strap of a weight cuff that sits over the ankle joint. If you don't have a weight cuffs at home, you can utilize a 1 kg salt packet and use a towel for wrapping it over the the lower leg.

It is best if the exercises are performed with both legs at the same time. Here is the exact method to perform this exercise.

Technique

Figure 14

1. The ideal starting point is lying flat on your back, with your hands on the side.

2. Then you can slowly raise your leg while keeping the knee straight.

3. Lift it up to not less than 30°.

4. Keep it on for 5 seconds then lower it slowly.

5. Repeat steps 2,3 as well as 4 for the other leg.

6. Repeat the exercise 10 minimum times in one session.

7. Start with a weight cuff using 0.5 kg weight. Gradually increase to 1 kg. Continue through 1.5 kg up to 2kg of weight.

The importance of exercise

The exercise can also be used to build the quadriceps muscle However, it is more resistant than static quadriceps workout. This is due to the fact that the individual is lifting their leg in opposition to gravity, and the the quadriceps muscles are working harder in order to perform this exercise.

Bullet points:

1. The distinction between static and dynamic quadriceps exercises is that the dynamic workout requires movement of the lower limbs around the hip joint.

2. It is important to note how the leg lifted and lowered.

3. It is more resistant in nature, and is more resistant to static quadriceps workout.

***

3: Strengthening the Adductors

This strengthening exercise is designed to increase the strength that runs along the inside of the lower thighs. The term used in medicine for the muscle is called the adductor muscle group. Before we get into the depths this figure outlines the process of exercise.

Start position

Figure 15

Position of the target

Figure 16

The description of the exercise to strengthen the adductor

This is a straightforward and effective exercise, but it is frequently ignored by rehabilitation specialists. Check out the image of a cushion that is placed between your legs. The arrow marks indicate that it's been compressed or more precisely compressing in between the legs.

A single pillow may not be enough to provide enough resistance. In this situation you can fold it up or you could use two pillows according to your needs.

So, what's the precise method?

Technique

1. Lay on your back and flat, keeping your knee bent in a position. Hands should be kept to the sides of your body.

2. Make sure you have a comfortable pillow between your thighs. The pillow should be

strong enough to permit sufficient pressure If not, then fold it in the center. There is the possibility of using two pillows at a time.

3. The pillow should be placed between your legs, hold it for 5 seconds, then let it go slowly. The most effective method is to count from 1 to 5 to hold the pillow for 5 seconds.

4. Repeat this process 30-40 times in one session.

The importance of the exercise

The purpose of this exercise is to build your hip muscles. Although it does not have an impact on the motion of the knee joint, it has an impact on the biomechanics of knee joint.

They are situated on the inside of the thigh. It serves an significant function in bringing about hip joint in adduction. joint.

Adduction is a motion of the body part toward the body. That is why it is known as an adductor hip set of muscles. They are a set of five muscles.

Bullet points:

1. Adductor muscles are located on the inside of the thigh.

2. It plays a vital role in moving the leg toward the body.

3. By placing a pillow between your knees and pressing them will result in the thigh moving inwards. This exercise can be designed to build the adductor muscle that runs along the side of your thigh.

***

4. Strengthening exercises for abductor

The name implies the abductor strengthening exercises are to build muscle that is opposite to the adductor muscle mentioned above.

The abductor muscle group is the most important muscle. Let's get started with these two pictures that illustrate the starting and goal positions during the training.

Starting position

Figure 17

The target posture

Figure 18

A description of how to perform the task

It is also a type of straight leg raising The only difference is that it's performed from a position that is side-lying. The leg that is done is kept at the highest point.

Let's suppose that you would like to work the left knee. Place the left leg on top of the other by lying side-to-side on the right side (as in the picture below).

Let's explore its strategy.

Technique

Figure 19

1. Lay down on your back (left or right).

2. In general the knee that is to be exercised must be maintained on top.

3. The knee below is held in a bent the position to give a wider base of support as well as good stabilization.

4. For instance, if you need to do the exercise on your right knee, you can lie down on your side and keep your left knee bent slightly.

5. Then, slowly lift the right leg, but no more than thirty degrees.

6. For 5 seconds, hold it and slowly lower it.

7. Repeat it at least 10 times in a single session.

The importance of this exercise

This is an abductor strength exercise that is designed to build the hip abductors group of muscles.

They are opposite to the muscles we discussed earlier and are the adductor muscle. They are muscles found in the adductor/outer compartment of the thigh. They are located on the outside of the thigh.

Figure 20 3 abductor figures

The actions of these muscles causes the abduction motion that occurs in the thigh. Abduction is when that the leg and thigh are able to move away from the body. The abductor muscle, which is strong, is essential for the normal biomechanics of knee joints.

Bullet points:

1. The muscle of the abductor is opposite to the adductor muscle.

2. They are located on the outside of your knee. Its purpose is to help move the leg to the outside.

3. The weight of the weight cuff can be used to increase the resistance load regularly. Start with adding 0.5 kg weight to one kilogram, 1.5 1 kg to up 2 kilograms of weight.

***

Five: Abductor short strength exercises

Start position

Figure 21

The target posture

Figure 22

The 5th exercise is a short abductor workout and is aimed at strengthening the abductor muscles of the short. They perform the same function as abductor, but they differ in hip position. The procedure is nearly the same as above but with a small variation as illustrated below.

Description of exercise

The beginning position of the exercise is nearly same as that of the prior exercise. The only difference is that the upper leg must be kept bent.

Another distinction is that unlike abductor strengthening exercises that are long in duration exercise, there is no straight leg raise. It's just a matter of raising the knee , keeping your feet in contact with the other.

This is the step-by step procedure.

Figure 23

Technique

1. Lay down on your back (leftor right) and the leg where the exercise must be done is maintained at the the top.

2. Keep both knees in a bent position, as illustrated in the image.

3. Slowly elevate the knee towards the top and ensure that your foot is maintained in contact with one the other.

4. Repeat it at least 30-40 times in one session.

Importance of the exercise

Both short and long abductors are found on the outside of the thigh, however they differ slightly in the way they operate.

Short abductor causes hip abduction movements in a hip flexion as well as mild knee flexion. The action can also affect the biomechanics of knee joint.

Bullet points:

1. Similar to long abductors. Short abductor muscles also appear on the outside of the thigh. It serves the same purpose as long abductors.

2. In reality this muscle group comes active when the hip joint is flexed halfway. When the hip is in this position, it's the abductor that is the most important part of the hip joint.

***

6: Knee Flexor Strengthening exercises

The back of the your thigh lies hamstring muscles and its contraction creates knee flexion. This is why it is referred to the knee flexor, and we will learn about its strength exercises. The image below provides an overview of the exercise.

Starting position

Figure 24

The target posture

Figure 25

Description of exercise

As you can see from the above illustration it's done in a prone position. Lying on the stomach is known as lying prone. It is possible to utilize a pillow to support your head as per your preference.

As always, it is important to keep knee in fully extended position. I'd like to note that it's a straight leg raise, but when you are lying down.

Here's the exact method.

Technique

Figure 26

1. Begin by lying straight on your stomach (prone to lie down).

2. Begin slowly to raise the leg in the manner shown in the image at a minimum of 30-degrees of angle. The knee must remain in a straight in a straight position.

3. For 5 seconds, hold it and then lower it slowly.

4. Repeat the same process with the other leg.

5. It is recommended to do at least 10 repetitions during a single session.

The importance of Exercise.

The muscles of this group are located in the flexor compartment of the thigh. It is located on the rear of our thigh. They are also known as hamstrings.

Hamstring muscles are large and strong muscles created by the combination consisting of 3 muscles. The muscles are semimembranosus, semitendinosus, and the biceps muscles.

Figure 27 Hanstring muscle

This action is crucial to knee flexion as well as hip extension. You can feel your back thigh to feel the bulkiness.

Bullet points:

1. In the preceding chapters, we have discussed muscles that is used to extend your knee (Quadriceps) Move the your leg backwards (Adductors) and then move legs outwards (Abductors).

2. The only muscle we're remaining with is the one that is responsible for the bending knee motion, also known as knee flexors.

3. This exercise can help build up the muscles in the back of the knee.

***

7: Quadriceps with closed loops strength

These are exercises performed on land and are as easy as they sound. This illustration provides clear images of the exercises. It is important to note that they are performed in a standing on the floor.

Starting posture and Target position

Figure 28

Description of exercise

It's often referred to as the semi-squat and we need to be able to bend our knees to the half-way point of doing squats.

The exercise is referred to as a closed-loop exercise since, when you are performing half squatting this exercise is performed in a loop

1. Forward bending with your lower back.

2. Bending forward at both hip joints.

3. Knee bends with both knees.

4. The movement of bending both at the ankles.

It's a land-based workout and the way to exercise is easy to learn, so let's discover the best way to exercise in a closed loop.

Technique

Figure 29

1. Keep your feet straight and your legs separated.

2. Then, bend your knees, as illustrated in the image It is important to note that bending is about halfway to the full sitting position. Return to standing gradually and slowly.

3. If this is a challenge for you, you can lean back towards the wall, and then proceed. In this way, you will get assistance and it is simple to do.

4. Repeat it at least 20 times.

The importance of this exercise

It's also an exercise to strengthen quadriceps muscles, a type of exercise that is dynamic and strengthens the muscles.

The main reason for this exercise is that it along with the quadriceps muscles and the muscle in behind of the thigh (hamstring muscle) and the muscle of the lower leg (calf muscle and anterior shin muscles) and the foot muscle is also included.

We've learned that the quadriceps muscle is responsible for an incline in the knee and hamstring contraction results in knee bend movement. Therefore, these exercises are essential to ensure stabilization of knee joints.

Bullet points

1. It is one of the quadriceps enlargement exercise.

2. It's distinct from other exercises for quadriceps. This being said, it's not restricted to a single joint, but rather multiple joints are involved.

3. All joint movements occur within the closed loop.

***

8: Calf muscle strengthening

The calf muscle's strength is equally important as muscles in thigh or knee. Because this muscle originates from the knee's posterior side this is a muscle that ought to not be neglected. It is easy to do as is shown in the figure below.

Start posture and Target posture

Figure 30

Description of exercise

The largest muscle at the back of the lower leg is the the calf muscle. This workout is designed to strengthen the muscle.

It is done in an upright position. It's extremely easy and efficient exercise. You can stand completely free of having to hold anything or utilize the support of a plinth, table or other object to increase stability and safety.

In the picture below in the image below, the model stands using the table's support. The procedure explains the step-by step procedure.

Technique

Figure 31

1. Straighten up and take the table's support or other items like a wall/ plinth, as shown in the picture.

2. It is also possible to do these exercises without help if you are in pain or your power allow it.

3. Slowly raise your body and place your feet on the floor You may notice a stretch in the muscles of the calf. Lower yourself slowly.

4. Repeat the exercise at least 20 times in one session.

The importance of exercise

The calf muscles is the most used muscle in our body. It has an important function in walking, standing and running.

Its actions cause the dorsiflexion movement (downward bend) on the sole of your foot. The in turn, the weakness of the calf muscles greatly impacts biomechanics of knees.

The Calf muscle is made up consisting of two muscles; soleus and gastrocnemius that originates from the medial and lateral side of the posterior knee. They are the bulky portion at the back of the lower leg. They join into tendoachilles, which inserts into the calcaneum bone.

The tendon that is hard just beneath the bulky calf muscle is tendoachilles. It is the strongest tendon in the human body.

While there are many other exercises to strengthen the calf muscles but this one is the best for the requirements to an OA knee patient.

Figure 32 Calf muscle

***

Exercises for stretching

In addition to the elements that contribute to stiff joints we covered earlier in this chapter there is one that is muscle tightness. Muscle "tightness" is a result of an increase in tension due to the active and passive mechanism.

In the passive, muscles may become shorter due to postural adaptation or scarring. Actively the muscles can shrink because of spasm or contraction. No matter the reason tightness can limit the range of motion and can cause a muscle imbalance (CURRENT concepts in MUSCLE STRETCHING to improve fitness and recovery 2012).

Stretching is an intervention that is commonly used during rehabilitation. The purpose of stretching is to increase the length of muscles and ROM and to help align collagen fibres while recovery of the capsule and muscle.

9: Knee posterior joint capsule stretching exercise

In the case of osteoarthritis knee, the joint capsule in the posterior side (back) of the knee usually gets stiff and tight. The stretching exercise is easy as shown in the illustration.

Figure 33

A description of how to perform the task

It is a vital exercise for stretching the posterior joint of your knee. For this stretch you will require an elastic band (theraband) or you could also make use of a bed or towel sheet based on the space available.

The long sitting position is the ideal starting point; keep the band of resistance as illustrated in the image below. The arrow indicates the direction of pull using both hands. While pulling, allow the ankle joint to bend to the point that you'll feel a stretch on the muscles of the calf.

The method of stretching is can be described as follows.

Technique

Figure 34

1. Sit in a long, sitting posture.

2. Get the towel or sheet and secure the foot using it. Hold the ends of the bedsheet using both hands as you pull. You can pull it till you sense the stretch behind the knee.

3. Pull it , hold the for 60 second then let it go.

4. Repeat the process two to three times in one session.

The significance of this exercise

Like all synovial joints the knee joint space is covered by the soft tissue structure known as the joint capsule.

As the process of resolving osteoarthritis progresses, it begins to alter the soft tissues surrounding the joint surface. In this case, the posterior portion of the joint capsule (behind the knee) is the most affected.

This causes stiffness and contracture of posterior capsule that manifests in discomfort behind the knee. In my clinical practice, I've noticed that when combined with the hot fomentation, stretching can work as a wonder.

Take note that if you are experiencing extreme pain in the back of your knee, you must not stretch until the pain eases. It is easy to manage pain by applying a balm for pain on the knee's back.

Within 10 minutes following the balm application After 10 minutes, apply heat treatment on the area to get the best results.

Bullet points:

1. The stiffness of the joint capsule that lies behind on the side of the knee may be the most common reason for pain in the back of the knee.

2. The tightness can also make it difficult from straightening fully the knee for some patients.

3. Extending it may prove advantageous in the fight against both issue.

Chapter 10: What Are The Factors That Can Contribute To Osteoarthritis?

The main cause in initial (idiopathic) osteoarthritis (OA) that is OA that is not a result from illness or injury, occurs due to the normal aging process of the joint.

1. The content of water in cartilage increases with age and the protein content of cartilage decreases due to biological processes.

2. Over time, the cartilage begins to lose its elasticity flake and create small pores in the skin.

3. In cases of severe osteoarthritis the cartilage cushions between the vertebrae of the joint have been completely destroyed and have disappeared.

4. Additionally, over time, the repeated use of an injured joint could mechanically cause irritation and agitation to the cartilage, leading to joint pain and swelling.

5. In the event that the cartilage cushion gone it causes increased friction between bones, causing irritation and restricted joint movement.

6. The inflammation of the cartilage can cause the formation of bone outgrowths (spurs which are also known as osteophytes) around joints due to the inflammation.

7. Osteoarthritis can be seen in multiple individuals from the same familia on very rare occasions, suggesting that the condition is an inherited (genetic) basis.

In the end, there is a consensus among experts that osteoarthritis can be result of a combination of the factors mentioned above that eventually result in an increase in the size of the cartilage in the joint that is affected.

Secondary osteoarthritis can be described as a form of osteoarthritis that occurs because of the presence of a different illness or medical health condition. There are a myriad of circumstances that can cause secondary osteoarthritis. These include:

Gout, diabetes, hemochromatosis and other hormonal issues are all linked to the risk of joint injury. The presence of obesity and repeated trauma or surgical procedures to joints can also be linked to higher risk.

The increased mechanical stress placed on the joint and, as a consequently, more wear and tear of the cartilage are the main causes of osteoarthritis among obese people. Obesity is by far the biggest risk factor in osteoarthritis of the knees, eclipsing the effects of age. Weightlifters are believed to be more prone to knee osteoarthritis as compared to the general population due in part to their body weight. It is thought that the constant injury in connective cartilage (ligaments bone, cartilage and cartilage) in footballers and soldiers causes an early knee arthritis for these people. It is interesting to note that long-distance runners don't appear to be more susceptible to osteoarthritis as suggested by studies on health.

The accumulation of crystals in cartilage could cause degeneration and osteoarthritis. These are both painful ailments. For people suffering from Gout, crystals from Uric Acid produce arthritis; for those suffering from pseudogout calcium pyrophosphate crystals trigger inflammation.

A small portion of people are born with joint structures that aren't properly formed (congenital anomalies) that are more vulnerable to wear and tear that results in the early degeneration and destruction of the joint cartilage. In the case of hip joint, the osteoarthritis of hip joints is usually caused by structural issues of the hip joints which are present from birth.

Early wear of cartilage and later osteoarthritis is also associated with hormone imbalances like the growth hormone deficiency and diabetes.

Osteoarthritis, as well as the degeneration of cartilage

A durable, rubbery material with a greater flexibility and soft as bone. It is a protective layer for joints within the body. The primary purpose of cartilage is to safeguard the edges of bones within the joint, while also allowing them to freely move against each other.

As a result of the breakdown of cartilage surface of these bones get pitted and rough. This can cause pain and discomfort within the joint and irritation to the tissues surrounding it. The damaged cartilage is not capable of self-healing. Because cartilage lacks blood vessels it is the reason.

When cartilage has worn off the cushioning buffer it creates does not exist anymore which allows bone-on-bone contact to take place. This could cause excruciating pain , as well as other symptoms associated to osteoarthritis.

The facts about knee pain that you need to be aware

Knee pain is a common problem that is caused by a myriad of reasons, ranging from accidents of a sudden nature to the effects from medical issues.

The knee joint can be restricted to a specific part of the knee or spread throughout all knee joints.

Physical limitations are often felt when knee pain is present.

A thorough physical exam will usually be needed to identify the root of the knee pain.

The cause of the problem is determined by the root for knee discomfort, proper treatment could be suggested.

In the case of knee pain, or even extreme joint pains, the outlook is generally good, however it might require surgery or other treatment in some instances.

What exactly is knee pain?

Inflammation and pain around the joint of knee (femur, tibia, and fibula) and in the patella (kneecap) or the ligaments, the tendons as well as the cartilage (meniscus) that surround the knee are the most frequent causes of knee pain. Apart from exercise and obesity knee pain, it can be caused due to the surrounding muscles and their movements, and it could result from other conditions (such as foot injuries). The knee pain can affect people from all ages. until the pain is extreme, home remedies can be beneficial.

What are the signs and signs of knee discomfort?

The location of knee pain can differ based the structure that is involved by the injury. A condition that is inflamed or infected could cause the entire knee to expand and become painful, while a ruptured meniscus or a fracture in a bone may only trigger symptoms in one location. Baker cysts are usually related to pain in the knee's back.

The intensity of joint pain could vary from a mild pain to a severe, painful throbbing pain that is excruciatingly debilitating.

A few of the other signs and symptoms that could be present when knee pain is present include:

It can be difficult to carry the weight or walk due to instabilities of knee. It becomes difficult walk upstairs or down due to ligament damage (sprain) and it's swelling and red. It is not possible for the knee to be stretched. it transfers weight to the other foot and knee; it's unstable.

What is the exact cause of knee discomfort?

Knee pain can be divided into 3 categories: arthritis or osteoarthritic and neuropathic.

fractured bone, tear in a ligament or a meniscal tear are some examples of injuries that are acute.

Medical issues like osteoarthritis, rheumatoid arthritis or infections can be possibilities.

Osteoarthritisand chondromalacia as well as Patellar disorders, bursitis, and tendinitis are all illnesses that are a result of long-term use or excessive usage.

A few of the most frequently-cited reasons for knee pain are listed in the following part of this article. This isn't an exhaustive list. Instead it provides a brief overview of some of the most common reasons for knee pain within every category mentioned prior to.

An acute knee injury is a type of injury that is quick to heal.

Bone fractures can occur in the event that a direct hit to the skeletal system causes the breaking of one or more knee bones. The result is typically the appearance of a painful and noticeable knee injury. Most minor knee fractures are extremely painful and many of them can affect the normal function of your knee (such as the kneecap fracture) and make it difficult to support an excessive amount of weight (such as tibial plate fracture). Every fracture should be evaluated by a physician as soon as possible. Many fractures require considerable force to be applied and a thorough exam is performed to determine if there are any other problems.

Ligament injuries The ACL (anterior cruciate ligament) injury is the most prevalent type injuries to ligaments. A ACL injury is usually sustained in a sport due to sudden stop and change in direction. The majority of injuries to the remaining ligaments (the posterior ligament for cruciate and the collateral ligament lateral as well as the medial collateral ligament) are located in the lower extremities.

Meniscus injuries Menisci (medial as well as lateral) comprise cartilage that acts as shock absorbers for the joints of knee. They can be triggered through a range of causes. Meniscus injuries can occur by a knee that is bent.

When the knee joint becomes dislocated, it's considered to be a medical emergency that requires immediate medical attention. A knee dislocation can result in that the supply of blood to your leg become impaired, in addition to other complications. A collision with an automobile usually results in injury to the knee, and this occurs when the knee hits the dashboard.

What medical conditions are at the root of knee discomfort?

Medical and medical issues and medicines

Rheumatoid Arthritis is an autoimmune condition that can be affecting any joint within the body. The most prevalent form of arthritis. It can cause significant pain and impairment as well as swelling in the event of not being treated quickly.

It is usually observed in the big toe but it could be affecting the knee as well. Gout is a type of arthritis which affects both the big toe as well as the knee. When gout is severe it can flare up and then becomes painful to the point of being excruciating. You can enjoy knees that are pain-free if there is no flare-up.

The condition known as Septic Arthritis (infectious arthritis) is a form of arthritis where the knee joint gets affected, leading to swelling, pain and fever. The use of antibiotics and drainage therapies must be administered as quickly as possible in this case.

Conditions that can be triggered by the use of drugs or alcohol for a long time

Patellar tendinitis refers to an swelling of the muscles which connect between the jointcap (patella) and the shinbone. It's caused by the overuse of the tendon (the bone in the leg's lower part). The condition is a long-lasting condition that is often experienced by those who exercise repeatedly and repeat the same exercise repeatedly (such as cyclists and runners).

It's caused through atrophy or strain under the knee (patella) at the point which connects to the thighbone. This can result to patellar pain disorder (femur). Patellofemoral painful syndrome an issue that affects runners and cyclists.

Osteoarthritis is a disease that is defined by the degeneration of cartilage in joints due to use and age.

The anterior knee is prone to pain. is caused by an inflammation in the bursa (fluid-filled sac) that is located in between the kneecap and its front. This is known as preatellar bursitis.

What are some potential risk factors to develop knee discomfort?

Biomechanics: The function of knee joints is complicated and is used frequently during the daytime. Small changes in the movement of the joint (leg-length discrepancy, changes in walking technique due to back problems) could cause injuries and discomfort in the event that the joint is not correctly adjusted.

Excessive weight: A lot of weight can put more strain over the knee joint which can result in injuries. Weight gain also increases the risk for developing osteoarthritis in the knee since it leads to cartilage degrading faster.

If cartilage is used up through repeated movements, for example, those observed during certain sports (such as skiing or running) or work-related situations (such prolonged time periods in which you knee) it can cause discomfort and break down.

When is the best time to visit your doctor if suffering from knee discomfort?

Any discomfort that doesn't diminish with rest, or doesn't improve in a short period of time should be evaluated by a physician whenever it is possible. There are additional knee-related symptoms and signs to look at: swelling inability bent, deformity inability to walk , or discomfort while walking, severe discomfort, and fever.

What tests and methods can be employed to determine if you are suffering from knee discomfort?

A doctor begins with questions about the overall health of the patient, and will then inquire regarding the cause of knee pain the patient is having (how many years, what is the duration and intense and what makes it more or less painful or worse, etc).

After that an exam of knee joints will be conducted. It will include stretching the knee through its entire range of motion checking the ligaments for stability, and then examining the knee for swelling and pain. It is often helpful to compare the results from the exam of your problematic knee with exam of opposite knee. In the event of determining a diagnosis and initiating treatment it is usually all that is required. Numerous studies have proven that an expert examination is more reliable than an X-ray scan in determining cancer.

In certain situations doctors may choose to perform further tests, including those listed below.

Radiologic tests

An X-ray is a simple procedure that can be used to identify fractures and degenerative changes to the joint of knees.

The MRI image of knee is utilized to examine the ligament's soft tissue for tears and cartilage injuries, as well as muscle injuries, as well as other ailments.

Blood tests

If arthritis, gout or any other medical issue is suspected, a doctor might request blood tests to confirmation.

Joint fluid is removed away from joints (arthrocentesis)

The elimination of a tiny amount of fluid from the knee joint could be an efficient method to diagnose certain ailments. The procedure is carried out by inserting a needle in the joint and removing the fluid out. This procedure is performed in a clean and safe environment. After the fluid is taken in, it is transferred to a lab to test and evaluate. This is particularly helpful when an infected knee joint is suspected, and also for identifying gout from other forms of arthritis. If there is an accumulation of fluid in the knee joint because of an injury that is severe or a traumatic event, draining the fluid could aid in easing the discomfort and decrease the chance of infection.

What types of physicians are experts in knee pain treatment?

Most times your primary physician will be able to assess and address knee discomfort. In the majority of cases an orthopedic surgeon should be consulted if knee pain requires surgery or if the cause of the discomfort requires additional analysis. For arthritis, gout or joint pain It is possible to talk to an orthopedic surgeon or a Rheumatologist.

What is the most effective way to manage knee discomfort?

It is as numerous kinds of knee discomfort as there are many types of diseases that can cause pain.

Medicines

It is possible to use medicines to solve a medical issue or to ease discomfort.

If you're using prescription painkillers that are anti-inflammatory to treat your knee pain regularly You should see your doctor to have the health evaluated.

Physical therapy is one type therapy that involves moving that the body.

Sessions of physical therapy that strengthen muscles that surround the knee could help in enhancing its stability and allow for most efficient mechanical motions. Engaging with a physical therapist can assist you in avoiding injuries, or even stop an injury from getting more severe.

Injections

For certain ailments, injecting medications directly into your knee could be beneficial. Corticosteroids and lubricants are two injections that are most commonly administered. Corticosteroids injections into the knee could help in treating knee arthritis as well as other knee pains. They typically need to be repeated every couple of months or more often. The same type of fluid as the fluid that is naturally present within your knee joint could be utilized to ease pain and improve mobility.

Exercise

Physical exercise can strengthen the muscles around your joints. This could aid in easing stiff joints. Try to get at least 20-30 minutes of activity every on a daily basis or at minimum, every day of the week. Select activities that are moderate and easy to perform, such as swimming or walking. Yoga and Tai Chi may aid in increasing joint flexibility and aid to treat joint pain.

Weight loss

Being overweight could put the pressure on your joints, which can cause discomfort. Weight loss can help in relieving the strain and reduce the pain by reducing inflammation. A healthy weight can decrease the chance of developing health problems like the cardiovascular and diabetes.

Not getting enough sleep

Relaxing your muscles can reduce inflammation and swelling in your muscles and joints. Don't put yourself down and don't try to push yourself too far. The ability to get enough rest at night can help you manage your pain more effectively.

The application of cold and heat treatment

Cold or heat therapy can be utilized to ease stiffness and muscle pain, according to your preferences. Apply the cold or hot compress to joints that are painful for 15 to 20 minutes several times throughout the day, for between 15 and 20 minutes in total.

As well as easing your symptoms, these actions can also help improve the quality of your life overall.

Exercises for people with osteoarthritis

Stretching exercises that are gentle can be beneficial to those who are suffering from osteoarthritis. This is especially true when you experience stiffness or pain in your hips, knees and lower back. You can improve flexibility as well as range of motion by stretching.

Like any fitness program make sure to consult your doctor prior to beginning the program to make sure you are taking the right course that meets your particular requirements.

If your physician is in agreement with stretching exercises, it is recommended to take these osteoarthritis exercises.

5 Exercises to Beat Osteoarthritis The Pain and Inflammation

The process of reducing osteoarthritis (OA) manifestations requires time and effort and could require some trial and trial and. Most treatment options consist of medications that ease swelling and pain. Don't ignore the benefits of exercise and physical activity can bring to your overall health. In addition to taking part in activities that are low impact like swimming and light walking, it is recommended to incorporate these five exercises for strengthening into your workout routine on a regular basis.

Training suggestions from trainers

Exercises that help you build strong muscles to help support joint pain and to increase your range of motion as well as mobility. They are listed below.

You can complete all the exercises without adding extra weight.

To increase the difficulty of your workout , as you gain the strength you need, try using a band of resistance as well as an ankle-weight.

Knee extensions are one type of exercise that requires you to extend the knees.

The quadriceps muscles you strengthen will prevent joint instability and give you more mobility and flexibility in daily activities.

Make sure your knee is close to the edge of your table or chair and then sit at your desk.

2. Straighten one leg towards the front by contracting your muscles in your thighs at the top of the movement.

3. You should extend your knee as long as it is able to be, and preferably over the 90-degree mark if it is possible.

4. This exercise should be done for 20 repetitions. Repeat the exercise for the opposite leg.

Leg raises when lying down

The quadriceps and hip flexors and the core muscles are all engaged in this exercise. It is especially beneficial to people suffering from osteoarthritis in the knees or hips and it can be done any time, laying on a bed or on the floor.

1. Place your feet flat on your back , with your knees bent with you feet resting on floor. 2.

Relax on the bed with your one leg stretched out to the side, your foot bent and your toes pointed towards the ceiling.

3. Move your leg up to the 45-degree mark, focusing on the muscles surrounding the side of

your thigh to raise your leg to a 45-degree angle.

4. Begin by counting one time at the highest point of the scale, and gradually lower the number. Focus on limiting the movement only one leg at a time while keeping your torso and hips as straight as is possible.

5. Keep going for 15 repetitions. Repeat the exercise with the opposite leg. Complete the three sets.

Squats against the wall using an stability ball

1. Put a huge stability ball against the wall. Lean against the ball with your back resting on the ball.

2. Keep your feet hip-width apart , and approximately 2 feet to the wall. Relax your shoulders and keep your eyes to your path ahead.

3. Slowly lower yourself to the position of a sit, but be careful not to lower your body further than a 90-degree angle.

4. Keep the ball in contact as you squeeze your glutes while returning to a standing position.

5. Do it 15 times and then take 15 minutes to rest, then repeat the process 3 times more.

Curls of the hamstrings when standing

1. Step back a bit and look towards either a chair or wall to maintain your equilibrium. Be sure that your feet are the width of your hips. Be sure to maintain a solid posture and focus your gaze ahead.

2. Move your foot towards your buttocks, while bent one leg to knee. While performing this

exercise, make sure you don't allow your body to swing between the two sides.

3. Continue steps 3 and four times each on the other side. Complete the three sets.

The hip abduction occurs when seated.

Sit on the edge your chair, back stretch as well as your feet and arms resting on the thighs of the chair you're sitting in.

2. Attach a band to your resistance, or a loop of resistance band around your thighs above your knees to give resistance.

3.) Move your knees to the side, pressing your glutes in the outer part to start the exercise.

4. Continue until you have completed 20 repetitions. Repeat until you have completed three sets.

Surgery is a viable option for curing and treating knee pain?

Surgery

Knee surgery can range from arthroscopic knee surgeries to total knee replacement, and everything between. When you undergo arthroscopic knee surgery small incisions as well as fiberoptic cameras are utilized to allow the surgeon to view inside the knee. It's a very common surgical procedure. A lot of injuries can be treated, and small pieces of bone that are loose or cartilage could remove by surgeons. This procedure can be performed in an outpatient setting.

When a knee replacement is a partial one surgeon replaces injured knee joints with metal and plastic components. Because only a fraction of the joint in question is repaired the time for recovery is shorter than the complete knee replacement.

Total knee replacement: This operation involves replacing the knee joint by the aid of an artificial joint.

There are many other options readily available.

Acupuncture is proving promising for treating knee pain, especially in those suffering from osteoarthritis. In studies studies on the effect of glucosamine as well as chondroitin supplements have not been consistent.

What are the best natural remedies you can use at home to relieve knee discomfort?

The over-the-counter pain relievers tend to be effective in helping to ease discomfort. If you are regularly taking these medications it is recommended to seek out a medical professional to get knee pain correctly diagnosed and to avoid the potential adverse effects from regular use of these medications.

It is the RICE mnemonic, that stands for Repose, Ice, Compression, and Elevation, is often helpful, especially for minor injuries:

Relax the joint and stop the things you typically perform that use your knee joints.

Ice The use of ice to reduce inflammation and pain may be beneficial.

Compression bandage: A compression bandage can help reduce swelling and help improve knee alignment. It should not be overly snug, and must be removed prior to going to sleep.

Maintaining your knee elevated can help reduce swelling and allow rest to your knee joints.

How can knee pain be a sign of a problem?

In most cases knee pain may ease without any reason being determined. The pain can get worse and then return in the future, possibly leading to more serious injuries or issues, based on the root reason. The majority of these ailments are chronic in nature and can cause discomfort or difficulty in walking due to.

Can you avoid knee discomfort?

Knee pain could be caused by a range of reasons. In turn, based on the root cause of the pain, a variety of strategies for pain relief are readily available. If the pain results from the overuse of jogging, jogging with soft surface or decreasing the duration of running can be beneficial. Knee injuries that are traumatizing could be avoided by avoiding direct injuries on the knee like wearing seatbelts. Weight loss can be beneficial for a range of kinds of knee discomfort.

Does it make sense that knee pain will be re-inflicted following treatment?

Knee pain can manifest it for a short period of time before it disappears. It could reappear several weeks or even months later. It is essential to have the knee in pain that is persistent to avoid further damage in the bone, cartilage or ligaments in the knee. The diagnosis can be determined by root causes of the discomfort.

In a lot of cases of knee pain, the latest surgical techniques allow you to relieve the symptoms and return to an active life.

Osteoarthritis at its worst

OA can be described as a degenerative condition that develops over five stages, which range from 0 to. The first stage (0) shows the normal joint in its simplest shape. Stage 4 represents the most severe manifestation of OA. Most people who suffer from OA do not progress until they reach stage 4. In most cases the disease is stabilized prior to reaching this stage.

Patients with severe OA suffer from significant or complete destruction of the cartilage some or all joints, which could be life-threatening. If bones rub against each another, it can result in extreme symptoms, such as the ones below.

The swelling and edema have been increasing. The amount of synovial fluid inside the joint could increase. The normal function of this fluid is to aid in reducing friction in motion. However, if used in large quantities it can cause swelling of joints. The presence of cartilage fragments in synovial fluid could further increase the discomfort and cause edema.

The intensity of pain has increased. It is possible to feel pain when you are exercising and even when you're laying down. In the course of the day you could be noticing an increase in your discomfort and also an increase in swelling in your joints , if you've used these joints frequently during the daytime.

The movement range has decreased. Due to the stiffness or discomfort in your joints, you might not be in a position to move as easily as you'd like to. This can make it harder to perform the duties of everyday life that were once part of your routine.

Instability of joints. Your joints might be less stable. Think about the scenario of someone suffering from osteoarthritis that is severe in their knees. They may experience locking (sudden absence of movement). If your knee becomes swollen and you are unable to move it, you could get injured or fall due to the.

There are other signs. The muscles are weakening, there are bone spurs and joint deformities can occur due to the continual wear and tear on the joint.

While the joint degeneration caused due to severe OA is irreparable, treatment can help ease the symptoms associated with the disease.

Osteoarthritis as opposed to. Rheumatoid Arthritis Which is the better choice?

While osteoarthritis (OA) along with Rheumatoid Arthritis (RA) are both afflicted with several of the same characteristics, they're completely distinct illnesses. OA causes debilitating disease and this implies it is more severe. condition gets worse as time passes. In contrast, RA is classified as an autoimmune disorder.

Patients with RA suffer from immune systems that mistake the lining of joints as a threat to the body, causing an immune system that attacks the joint. Synovium, also known as the synovium membrane is spongy lining which is filled with synovial fluid. It is located between joints. When the immune system starts attacking the joint fluid builds up within the joint, creating stiffness, pain as well as inflammation, edema, and swelling in addition to other signs.

Speak to your doctor is the best way to go when you're not certain what kind of arthritis you suffer from. However, you can investigate.

The diet to treat osteoarthritis

There aren't any negative side effects of eating healthy, however when you suffer from osteoarthritis, diet and nutrition are important.

Maintaining your weight in a reasonable range can reduce the pressure that is that is put on your joints which is good for.

There is evidence that suggests that some forms of OA like osteoarthritis of knees, could respond well to a diet high in flavonoids. They are substances found in vegetables and fruits, according to research. Additionally the antioxidants in a wide variety of fruits and vegetables might be able to aid in fighting free radicals triggered through inflammation. Free radicals are chemical compounds which have the potential to cause harm to cells.

In order to reduce swelling and inflammation A high-quality diet could provide relief from the signs of osteoarthritis. Consuming foods that are high in the following nutrients could be beneficial

Vitamin C and vitamin D are important nutrients.

beta-carotene

EPA and DHA are omega-3 fatty acids.

Furthermore to this, increasing the amount of foods with anti-inflammatory properties can be beneficial.

How to eat right if You Are Suffering from Osteoarthritis at the Knee

Osteoarthritis (OA) that affects the knee is a condition that occurs when cartilage in the joint gets worn out, causing bone to degrade. The knee joint is affected by OA. It's an autoimmune disorder that affects knee joints. Apart from the injury to tissues, you'll probably experience discomfort and swelling due to the injury.

Certain dietary options can aid in the treatment and prevention of joint pain.

This article will explain the foods you can eat to increase your health and the joint of your knees as well as how you can do it.

What role do food items play in OA

Your eating habits and the food you consume could influence the development of osteoarthritis.

According to researchers according to scientists, when inflammation is present the body produces chemicals known as free radicals which can be detrimental on the body. Free radicals form within the body because from exposure to toxic substances or natural processes, like inflammation and infection.

Oxidative stress is a condition that occurs when an excess amount of free radicals build up. Oxidative stress could cause tissue and cell injury throughout the body including the brain.

Additionally, damage to the synovium or cartilage which both aid in the cushioning of knee joints could be a possibility. Oxidative stress could cause the onset of inflammation that is not previously present.

Antioxidants are substances that can help protect the body from damaging free radicals. They are found naturally within the body and can be sourced them through plant-based foods and drinks.

The precise mechanism through which oxygenative stress and free radicals create OA isn't known, but certain studies have suggested that antioxidant supplements could prove beneficial.

A diet that permits you to maintain a healthy weight will help in managing arthritis of knee.

Foods to eat

A wide range of nutrients could help in improving joint health and decreasing inflammation.

Include these items in your diet can help to in preventing or slowing the progression of osteoarthritis

Eat lots of vegetables and fruits and are rich in antioxidants.

Dairy products with low-fat content that are rich in calcium and vitamin D and nutritious oils like olive oils that are extra-virgin olive are suggested.

These are the items included in the anti-inflammatory diet.

Foods to avoid

Certain foods can make it more likely that you will develop an oxidative stress.

The following food items have the potential for having this impact:

foods that have been highly processed

food items that are loaded with sugar and unhealthy fats such as saturated fats and trans fats are deemed to be harmful.

Foods with crimson colors

Consuming these foods may increase levels of inflammation in your body.

Vitamin C acts as a potent antioxidant.

Vitamin C is an important nutrient, and also functions in the role of an antioxidant. It is needed by your body to support the creation of cartilage which is a protective layer for bones in the knee joint. It could also aid in the elimination from free radicals.

An adequate consumption of Vitamin C could help in preventing the development in OA symptoms.

Incorporate these items into your shopping cart

Papaya, guava and pineapple are all examples of tropical fruit.

A sense of caution should be taken when eating citrus fruits like grapefruit and oranges. Other fruits and veggies to be consumed include cantaloupe the kiwi, strawberries, and raspberries. Other veggies include cruciferous ones (such as broccoli, cauliflower and the kale).

Vitamin D and calcium are both important.

The findings of a few researchers have suggested that vitamin D could help in the treatment or prevention of osteoarthritis. However the evidence is not conclusive.

A study that was published in the year 2019 did not find any evidence that vitamin D could help in reducing the progress of osteoarthritis however, it did suggest it might be beneficial in relieving joint pain for those with low blood levels of vitamin D.

A new research project

In a research conducted through Trusted Source, individuals with high levels of calcium in their blood showed lower amounts of osteoarthritis damages.

Vitamin D assists with the absorption process of calcium in the body. Consuming foods that are high in these nutrients could be beneficial in a small way.

Vitamin D can be obtained through controlled exposure to sunlight and certain food items which are rich in vitamin D can be absorbed through eating them.

The foods that are rich in calcium, vitamin D as well as all three ingredients are:

seafood, including cod and wild-caught salmon as well as sardines as well as shrimp, canned seafood like tuna; fortified milk and dairy products as well as other products

eggs

Yogurt, leafy green vegetables and more

Other food items that contain or are supplemented with calcium or vitamin D are:

orange juice, breakfast cereals tofu and breakfast cereals are great choices.

In the absence of evidence to suggest that vitamin D supplements could help in the treatment of osteoarthritis, the current guidelines do not recommend using vitamin D supplements for this condition.

Always consult your doctor prior to using any supplements, since certain supplements might not be suitable for all to use.

Carotene (beta carotene)

Additionally, beta carotene which is an extremely potent antioxidant. it's easy to identify because it is the reason behind the vibrant orange hue of vegetables and fruits like carrots, which makes them appear distinct. Beta carotene is an effective antioxidant that's good for your eyes, skin and hair.

Some other excellent resources include:

vegetables that contain cruciferous elements like Brussels sproutsand collards mustard greens, and chard as well as leafy greens like romaine lettuce and sweet potatoes, cantaloupe, winter squash; peppermint, apricots, parsley tomatoes; asparagus; and peppermint

Omega-3 Fatty Acids are vital to maintain healthy well-being.

In a few studies it has been suggested that the consumption of higher levels of omega-3 fats over omega-6 fatty acids can aid in preventing osteoarthritis.

Below are some suggestions for striking the perfect balance:

The use of omega-3 fatty acids like olive oil, in salad dressings, cooking, and cooking is recommended.

Consuming fatty fish two times a week and limiting the consumption of red meat and other animal-based foods

A cup of seeds or nuts daily can help reduce inflammation within the body through reducing the production of cytokines as well as enzymes which break down cartilage.

These foods provide great source of omega-3 fats

Salmon is fresh, wild or tinned is a delight. Mahing and Herring are both readily available, however there is no king mackerel.

Salves, anchovies and rainbow trout Pacific oysters and eggs enhanced with omega-3 fat acids (ground flaxseed and flaxseed oils) as well as walnuts and many other nuts

Omega-6 fatty acids are found in the following food items:

Meat and eggs, poultry, grains, seeds and nuts as well as some vegetable oils can be some examples of the staple food items.

According to the current guidelines According to current guidelines, taking supplements containing fish oil is not advised since there is no evidence to suggest that they have any benefit.

Bioflavonoids

Antioxidants, in the form bioflavonoids, like quercetin and anthocyanidins are also available.

Quercetin is a natural anti-inflammatory agent and animal studies suggest the possibility of using it in treating osteoarthritis in the coming years.

These are great quercetin sources:

Onions (red yellow, red, and white) Kale (leeks) cherries tomatoes (broccoli) Blueberries (black currants) and lingonberries (cocoa powder) (cocoa powder), Green tea (green tea leaves) Apricots (with skin) Apples with skins

Spices

Certain spices contain ingredients which have anti-inflammatory properties too. Both turmeric and ginger can be considered to be two potent natural cures.

30 people who ingested 1 milligram of powdered ginger daily day for eight weeks experienced an improvement in knee pain and also improvement in mobility and overall well-being as per a tiny study.

Check out these recipes to incorporate ginger into your diet:

Fresh ginger can be added for stir-fries, salad dressings, or to make with grating.

Ginger tea is made by steeping ginger pieces in hot water.

Muffins that are made from high-fiber, low-fat ingredients are enriched by the powdered ginger.

Curries, biscuits, cakes and apple dishes all benefit by the addition of freshly-ground or powdered ginger.

Turmeric can be described as one of the Asian spice that has a mustard-yellow color and is the main ingredient of yellow curry. It's mostly made up of curcumin.

A recent study revealed that eating around 1 g curcumin every day for between 8 and 12 weeks could help to reduce inflammation and pain that is caused by osteoarthritis.

The supplements and goods made from turmeric can be purchased online. Always consult your physician prior to using any supplements to make sure they are safe to take.

Chapter 11: What Are The Signs Of Arthritis?

Pain If you are suffering from knee pain, it could be coming out of your knee. It is important to consult your doctor since knee pain could be caused to other areas in your body. There are many different causes of knee pain that are not related to arthritis. Some of these are more serious and can even lead to death.

However, people who are recognized as having knee arthritis are likely to suffer from discomfort. The pain can start at any time, but typically the arthritis-related pain will develop gradually. The pain at first may appear only when you first get out of bed or have been sitting inactive for a certain amount of duration.

In the near future, you could begin to feel pain as you walk up and down steps. Soon you could experience discomfort when walking on flat surfaces. If the damage does not stop then you could experience discomfort even when you are asleep frequently waking you multiple times throughout the night.

A lot of my patients inform me that knee pain was more intense during colder weather.

Stiffness is when your knee is unable to produce enough lubricant, it becomes more difficult to bend it completely. It is possible that you're in a position where you cannot bend your knee when you get up stairs or engage in other things. In the end, simple daily tasks like walking can become difficult.

Swelling - fluid may develop around your knee. The fluid may also develop in your knee joint - it's known as an effusion. A doctor will determine if you've an effusion. The fluid from knee effusions is not worth the effort since it's not a reliable fluid. If you locate a physician within your vicinity who treats knee arthritis, he/she might suggest the draining of that fluid.

Crepitus sounds are the sound that occurs when the cartilage in your knee rubs. The lack of lubrication indicates that the cartilages don't move effortlessly, and that's why cartilage wears off each when you move your knee in a bent position to take one step.

Locking, collapse When the root of the arthritis is not addressed, then the muscles surrounding the knee are beginning to shrink. This could cause instability. If your knee is locked or collapses , you run the risk of causing further injury.

What are the advantages that come from Knee Replacement Surgery?

It is possible that taking out the knee joint that is arthritic in exchange for a new joint will reduce stiffness and pain, and thus enhance your life quality. The purpose in knee replacement surgeries is to let you to resume activities you've been unable take pleasure in.

The majority of patients who undergo the First Total Knee Replacement surgery are happy.

In a review of 17 different studies in 2012, the British Medical Journal in 2012 found that 36% of those who decided to undergo knee surgery less or no better than before.

Even after 12 months from their surgery, the patients complained that they :

* The pain didn't improve following knee replacement surgery or even got much worse. A lot of people end up taking addictive painkillers.

* Their mobility was diminished. They were unable to walk, difficult to sit down and much more difficult to climb the stairs. They could not dance or garden, bowl or engage in other sports, and it even affected their sexual life.

As is to be expected, a large percentage of patients felt anxious or depressed for a period of 12 months after knee replacement surgery.

These problems are often none to do with technological difficulties caused by the procedure or any negligence or negligence of the doctor. The high rate of failure in knee replacement surgery was observed in a variety of centers.

What are the potential risks associated with Knee Replacement Surgery?

The top ten reasons those who've had one knee replacement do not want to get the second knee replaced:

* Failure as high as 36% of patients have the same pain or even worse

* inflammation of the wound, or even an infected the artificial joint. This can be catastrophic and require removal of the joint infected or life-long antibiotics

* excessive loss of blood (severe enough to require a the transfusion of blood);

* Blood clot (DVT / Deep Vein Thombosis) is especially hazardous, particularly when the blood clot inside the leg suddenly ruptures and travels to the lung and can result in immediate death.

* wound breakdown

* fractures caused by surgery

* reaction to anaesthetic, ranging from a rash of nausea to an allergy, and eventually death

* Joints that are unstable or loose could require additional surgery to repair;

* heart, respiratory, kidney problems

* death .25%

Is There a Safer, More Effective Method?

Yes.

For certain types of people.

There is hope, as there may be a viable alternative for surgery should you be eligible. Since you might be able replace the joint fluid.

Like a car that is getting old and requires more oil, when your knee joints age, they will require more lubrication in order to prevent any further wear and wear and tear. It's similar to refilling and topping up the engine oil that is vital to your vehicle every six months to avoid any further damage, stop the wear and tear and make your knee to function more efficiently and pain-free.

Are you able to see how this could help you?

What could this mean for your way of life?

Today, there are many products available out there. However, the most important thing is to locate the right doctor in your area in the globe who

* is a specialist in knee injections (i.e. injects more than 50 times each week) since the safety and effectiveness are related to the amount of injections they perform as well as

* who utilizes specialized equipment for ultrasound or any other type of imaging device because they can actually see the NEEDLE and guide the needle into the correct spot for YOU. A lot (if not all) injectors fail due to the fact that the surgeon or doctor does not use ultrasound.

However, if you come across an acupuncturist who gives many knee injections per day and utilizes ultrasound, you should:

* the odds of getting there are 79.7 percent or more; and

* the chance of complications is lower than one percent

If the injections are done correctly, there are three primary reasons for why this treatment works extremely well:

1. Because the product offers an oily lubrication for an inside part of your knee joint and makes it less painful for you and

2. This stimulates your synovial cells and you start making more joint fluid. This means that you'll be happier and pain-free for longer.

3. The fluid can also act in the capacity of a shock-absorbing agent. It gives the user less pain when they dance, stand, walk and play bowls, golf or any other activities of the day.

Chapter 12: What Is Osteoarthritis Knee?

Osteoarthritis (OA) knee, also known as OA is a knee pain that can develop spontaneously as you age. It causes your knee to appear swelling and can make everyday activities such as walking, climbing stairs or squatting, as well as the cross-leg sitting experience. If the condition is severe it is possible to in bed.

To fully understand osteoarthritis, you must first understand the terminology used to describe it. The term"osteoarthritis" actually the combination of two words "osteo" as well as "arthritis".

Osteo refers to bone or is related to bone, and arthritis refers to joint inflammation. In the public health sector arthritis is a general term that refers to the more than 100 illnesses or conditions that adversely affect joints, the tissue surrounding joints, as well as other connective tissue(Lespasio and others.).

When knee joint inflammation (or the other joints) results from the process of degenerative aging or weight, as well as repeated microtrauma resulting from a specific positions, leading to wear and tear on the cartilage as well as the bone of the knee, it is known as Osteoarthritis (OA) knee.

So, how do be defined OA knee?

Osteoarthritis knee is a degenerative joint disease that results in gradual but irreparable damage to the smooth cartilage in the knee joint. It gets rough and worn away, leading to discomforting friction on the cartilage surfaces.

The knee joint's surface is smooth as it is covered by a the smooth line of cartilage to allow to allow for smooth and non-slip movement. In OA the surface is eroded and this is accompanied by an increase in wear and tear of the joint as a result of the effects of weight, age, and joint trauma caused by repetitive motions particularly the squatting position and kneeling(Heidari).

In order to understand this, we need to know a bit about the anatomy of the regular knee joint.

Anatomy of the knee joint

The knee joint can be a movable hinge joint which allows the user to move with great ease. The human body generally consists of two kinds of joints. One is immovable, and the other is a moveable. Like the name implies, the joints that move allow movement, and have a different anatomy from an immovable joint.

Figure 1 Anatomy of knee joint

The joint with a movable motion is surrounded by a capsule that creates an area of joint between the two surfaces of articulation. It is full of body fluids and plays a crucial function in acting as fluids.

The fluid used to lubricate the body is known as synovial fluid, and that is the reason why joints that move are also referred to as synovial joints. It is possible to compare this fluid to the lubricating fluid is used in automobiles and bicycles for seamless and frictionless motion of wheels.

The surface of the joint is the of the line which is involved in formation of the joint, and two surface articulars form the joint.

When a joint is normal the two surfaces of the articular (surface of bone that participates in the formation of joint) are smooth as they are laminated with cartilage. Smooth enough to permit smooth, pain-free motion of joints. Under cartilage is subchondral bone.

What exactly causes osteoarthritis?

Joint changes occur in OA knee

In the case of osteoarthritis, the joint surface is eroded and rough. It is possible to see an illustration showing a typical joint as well as one with osteoarthritic arthritis.

When someone suffering from OA knee is walking on a rough surface, it gets in contact with the knee and creates friction. Yes, friction causes joint movement to become painful.

In the process, swelling can develop around it, and, if it is not dealt with properly the friction that continues to build reduces the joint.

2. Normal knee vs. OA knee

A clinical manifestation of knee pain due to osteoarthritis

In my 11-year working in physiotherapy, I've witnessed a variety of OA knee injuries. The most frequent complaint that they have is knee pain while walking or stair climbs.

If they lie down on the ground, it can be difficult to stand up and even getting to a standing position after lying on the bed can be difficult.

In the morning, following sitting for a long time, or following a prolonged sleep are common. As time passes, the painful symptoms are more common in the evening, or during sleep during the night(Lespasio and others.).

Let's look at the symptoms in detail.

1. The onset of pain is often insidious and occurs when you perform activities that require weight bearing over the knee. These include activities like walking or squatting, stair climbing (eg. using the Indian method of toilet) and sitting cross-legged.

2. Stiffness and pain in the morning: Patients will experience stiffness and pain in the knee during the early morning. It may ease by moving and will improve as the day progresses.

3. Crepitus: Crepitus is a crackling sound that is released out of joint while the joint is moving. It is very common in OA knee. Patients frequently complain of a crackling sound emanating of the knee when they perform the knee's movements.

4. Boney enlargement and articular degeneration can be seen on the X-Ray.

***

The stages of OA knee

We have mentioned in our introduction that osteoarthritis is degenerative and, based on the extent of the degeneration of OA knee, we can classify it into stages. Beginning at the beginning stage, through intermediate to the late stage, the degeneration is more severe and irreparable.

Doctors employ X-ray radiological examination to evaluate the changes. The joint's degeneration is visible on an X-ray image. Based on these radiological results, Kellgren as well as Bier in 1957, first classified the degree the severity OA(KELLGREN and LAWRENCE).

This chapter we'll examine this gradation and try to understand it from the beginning stage intermediate stage, the late stage.

Similar to earlier surveys (Kellgren and Lawrence 1952, and Lawrence in 1955) osteoarthrosis was classified into five classes according to follows(Kohn and Lawrence, 1952; Lawrence, 1955).):

* N/A (0)

"Doubtful" (1)

* Minimum (2)

Moderate (3)

* Extreme (4)

The grade 0 is an absolute absence of changes in x-rays of OA and we should therefore ignore this grade. The Grades 1 and 2 of OA are are in our opinion are definitely present even although they are of a lesser degree, which is why we should classify these two grades as the first phase of classification.

Figure 3: The stages of OA knee

Also, let's put Grade 3 under mid-stage and Grade 4 under the late stage.

In the next chapter, we will attempt to comprehend the degenerative changes observed in these grades and how they manifest through symptoms and signs.

We'll start our discussion by discussing the the early stage of OA knee.

The beginning stages OA knee

The initial stage is the beginning phase of OA knee. It is when a patient first experiences minor knee discomfort. There is a growing awareness of the importance of discovering the beginning stages of degenerative process in the knee joint osteoarthritis (OA) that is the stage of disease during which there is still a potential for regenerative capacity in the cartilage articular which will be lost permanently when the disease progresses to advanced stage.

The patient feels discomfort only when in a certain posture of foot and leg when standing or climbing stairs.

The pain is so minimal that the sufferer often ignores the issue by linking it to their daily routine.

Figure 4 The early stage of OA knee

We have placed in Kellgren-Lawrence (KL) grades 1 and 2 in this stage, let's discover what changes in the knee joint occur in this stage of OA knee.

There is some doubt about the shrinking in joint space.

There is a possibility of osteophytes.

In normal circumstances, there is a space between joints, and as we've examined, it is full of synovial fluid. In OA knee the joint space tends to shrink. At this phase it seems to have begun to shrink, but it's not certain.

Additionally also, the X-Ray study shows that the osteophytes begin to show up along joints.

They are tiny bony projections that restrict joint's motion and cause pain when the joint is moved.

Intermediate stage

Intermediate stage is the middle stage between the beginning stage and the end stage. We can examine the character of this stage as Grade 3 in the kellgren Lawrence method.

The grade III Kellgren Lawrence is characterised by

1. Multiple osteophytes

2. A definitive joint space narrowing

3. Sclerosis can be seen as a rise in white areas of joint's bone along the joint's marginand

4. Possible bony malformation.

Figure 5: Intermediate stage

When the process of wear and tear alters the initial stage of OA knees, the joint enters an intermediate phase. In this stage , the joint space shrinks further and it becomes more difficult to detect. The increased bone formation or osteophytes growth on the joint's lips hinders joint motion due to stiffness and pain.

Late stage

The most painful and serious stage, there's significant reduction in joint space. The joint space is so small that even the articular face becomes in contact with each the other.

Figure 6: Late stage

The cartilage is nearly gone and the smooth surface of the joint gets rough.

It is distinguished by

1. Large osteophytes

2. The joint space is narrowed by a mark,

3. Severe Sclerosis, and

4. A bony deformity is definitely present.

The late stage of OA pain can lead to anxiety and anxiety, depression, fear of movement and a negative psychological outlook. Fear of moving can make it difficult to participate in exercises and social gatherings, leading to more social and physical marginalization (Kevin Vincent, 2012). Vincent 2012).

***

How do you manage OA knee discomfort

There is no treatment for osteoarthritis knee , and usually people live for about 30 years suffering from this condition. However, we can take care of it and stop beginning stages from becoming intermediate or later stage. If we do not stop the progression, we could at least slow the process of degrading.

Most medical treatment is for symptomatic reasons and can result in temporary relief of symptoms without taking into account of the risk over time. In contrast, those with OA knees Physical Therapy, as well as lifestyle counseling are not utilized as much, whereas the use of pain medications is increased(Khoja and colleagues.).

There is ample research evidence to establish the effectiveness of lifestyle changes such as exercise and weight loss and should be a priority for all patients due to the small danger of harm. The use of NSAIDs should be minimized to avoid gastrointestinal complications(Charlesworth et al.).

This book we'll discuss the treatment of osteoarthritis knee in the following categories:

1. Exercises for knee rehabilitation.

2. Pain management tips.

3. Lifestyle modification.

In the subsequent sections, we'll place an emphasis on knee rehabilitation exercises. Along with it , we'll examine lifestyle changes which are crucial to the overall efficiency of exercises. I've chosen the exercises that I normally give to my patients at the physiotherapy center, and have seen the positive results. Each exercise thoroughly, focusing on aspects like its effects the anatomy, and what it means.

Alongside this we will also go over some of the top and effective techniques to alleviate the pain-related symptoms.

It is important to note that while the methods for relieving pain can provide temporary relief. However, for lasting effect one has to concentrate on exercising and lifestyle adjustments. But, it can encourage you to keep going in the exercise. In the end, nobody wants to exercise with pain, does it?

This also highlights an important point that certain exercises may not be effective for various phases in OA knee. In reality, many exercises are extremely difficult to perform at the end of the stage, and could even worsen the symptoms.

To accomplish this I have organized the book in a way that we begin by covering the basics of exercises. In the next chapter, we will be able to understand what exercises should be done in what stage, and how to introduce slight variations (like the inclusion to the weight) to meet the needs of that specific stage.

Let's begin with knee exercises for rehabilitation.

***

Exercises to help knees recover

In the long-term management in the future of OA knees, conservative treatment is the most preferred method of treatment. But, while the use of conservative treatments is recommended for patients who have advanced to intermediate stages OA that affects the knee. However, later stage might require surgery. However, research supports the idea that exercise during the late stage could aid in avoiding surgery and is often performed as a pre-operative treatment plan.

Due to knee pain the exercises of the patient diminish, which leads to secondary muscle weakening around knee. The research has also proven that weakness in muscles (quadriceps muscles, specifically) is one of the causes for osteoarthritis knee(Slemenda and co.) and forming the vicious cycle of weakness of the quadriceps as well as OA joint pain.

Because weakness in muscles is associated with physical and pain and is a factor in the progress of the disease(Slemenda and colleagues.) for patients suffering from OA at the knee. strengthening of muscles is a crucial aspect in the cases of OA.

However, knee exercises include some stretching exercises. The best part is that the exercises can be done at home. I've experienced the patient's experience that a basic regimen of quadriceps exercises at home will significantly reduce symptoms of knee joint pain, as reported by the patient and function(O'Reilly and others.).

It's a good idea to review the anatomical foundations of the muscles in the area of the knee joint to get an improved understanding of the function of exercises for this type of discomfort.

Anatomy of knee joint muscles

The knee joint's motion is controlled by a variety of muscles and muscle groups surrounding the knee and thigh. These muscles cause an extension and bend of the knee.

The muscles or group of muscles are found all over the thighs. Examine your thigh, note its weight, this is due to the weight of the muscles. They're located on the back, front and sides of the the thigh as seen in the image below.

Figure 7

These muscles are

1. In front Quadriceps muscle.

2. In the inner side, there is an Adductor group of muscle.

3. The outer side of the Abductor Group of muscle.

4. Behind: knee flexors section of muscle.

Every muscle plays a specific role , and when used in a coordinated manner they are responsible for the movement within the joint of knees.

The quadriceps muscles in the front of the thigh is the one responsible to extend the knee (straightening) movement. The reverse action i.e. the knee bends caused by the action of the muscle on the side of Thigh (hamstring).

The role of the adductor muscles (on the inner side of the thigh) and abductor muscles groups is moving our legs towards the body and away from it and vice versa. While, their actions do create motion in the knee joint, they play a significant role in knee biomechanics.

The reason for this is that in OA knee, the muscles are weak because of the long-term inactivity or diminished mobility. This is caused by discomfort and impairment. A weak muscle is not capable of securing the joint, results in a change in the normal biomechanics and increased stress on the cartilage of the articular region.

It is therefore essential to strengthen the muscles of the knee joint with strengthening exercises. In the coming chapters, we will discuss the intricacies of each muscle anatomy and ways we can improve it in a particular way.

***

***

Pain management tips

If you're regular exercising you may experience occasionally a bout of intense acute discomfort. If this happens, don't be concerned It's perfectly normal for it to occur during exercises. Instead of despairing it is essential to continue with the exercises.

The pain can be controlled with simple home-based tips and safeguards, for which you will require the right details. To do this, apply any balm for pain (ointment) to apply it over the knee. It should be left for around 10 minutes.

Within 10 mins, apply the knee with a heat treatment. The treatment could be administered with two methods. Select the one that is most suitable for you.

It is possible to give it the following methods:

1. Hot pads (hot water bag/hot pads).

2. Infrared lamps.

I would recommend the Infra-Red lamp in place of hot pads. It has more penetrating power and is more efficient.

Braces for knees

What are the reasons why knee caps (braces) are important to have? It is essential to strengthen muscles in order to lessen the load (offloading weight) on the joint of knee. Although muscle plays a crucial part in the offloading of knee joints, there are times when it will require strengthening. This can be achieved through braces.

Braces that are used to support the knee is often referred to as the knee cap. Braces for knees can come in two varieties. They are used depending on the severity of the pain.

Two types of knee braces are

1. Simply knee caps.

2. Braces for knees with hinged edges.

For less pain, a basic kneecap is suggested. For more severe instances the hinged brace will be the most appropriate choice.

A knee brace that is hinged

A typical knee cap

***

Lifestyle modification

The current treatment method places lifestyle changes at the top of the list over the use of drugs. Research has also shown that exercise(O'Reilly and co.) and lifestyle changes can lead to an improvement in health and quality of your life.

The most crucial element of lifestyle modifications is exercise and weight control. While exercise is a viable lifestyle change, recent studies suggest that combining exercise and losing weight through diet is superior than implementing both interventions on their own for obese or overweight individuals who suffer from knee OA(Focht).

Exercises

The entire book is focused on exercises. But, the exercises we have went over are specific to knee exercises. Studies have also shown that hydrotherapy, aerobics cycling and even dancing aid to improve the quality of life for OA knee patient.

Hydrotherapy has also been proven to be beneficial for osteoarthritis knee. A Brazilian study of women with OA knee showed that a planned six-week program of hydrotherapy with an educational plan led to more improvement in performance and pain in the short-term as compared to an education program alone(Dias and colleagues.).

Recommendations for exercises in the hydrotherapy

Exercises in hydrotherapy are simple and anyone can do it. It's done in the swimming pool . Water reaching up to waist level. is suggested.

The majority of the land-based exercises we talked about in this book are an element of these exercises with the sole different is that it is carried out in the water. The theory behind hydrotherapy is it provides buoyancy force to the joints, which makes the exercises more comfortable for the knee suffering from pain.

These exercises include:

* Standing on toes.

* Walking.

* Semi-squats

* Step-up

* Single leg standing.

* Knee bent when standing.

Standing on toes

Grab the bar's support or the edge of the swimming the pool, and then stand on toes.

Semi-squat

Single leg standing

Do a single leg stand for at least 10 seconds. Repeat the exercise on the opposite side.

Step-up

Walking

The sport of cycling can help knee hurt

Many of you are already doing it, and research(Salacinski and co.) has also proven that static cycling enhances your activity life and overall level of living.

Cycling could be thought of as an alternative option for those suffering from knee OA. A US study revealed that low-intensity cycling is more effective than high-intensity cycling for improving gait and function as well as reducing pain and improving aerobic capacity(Mangione and co.).

Let's look at the specifics of this study for more understanding.

A controlled trial randomized to a group of participants was conducted, where 39 adults with a mean age of 71 years were recruited for the study with complains of knee pain, and diagnosis of OA.

Participants were randomly allocated to a high-intensity (70 percent HRR heart rate) or a low-intensity (40 percent HRR) exercise group for 10 weeks of stationary cycling.

Participants cycled for about 25 minutes, 3 times a week. Prior to and following the exercise program, they took The Arthritis-Inflicted Measurement Scale (scale that measures arthritis pain) to evaluate the overall level of pain.

They were also evaluated for the quality of the actions:

1. Chair rise,

2. 6-minute walk test

3. Gait and

4. Exercise treadmill tests that have been graded.

The severe pains were reported every day by using an analog scale that was visible and McMaster, Western Ontario and McMaster.

Results: The analysis showed that participants from both groups had significantly better results when they were given a timed rise of the chair during the six-minute walk test, across a different speeds of walking.

Significant improvements were observed in the overall pain relief and increase in the capacity to exercise. No differences between groups were found. Reports of pain on a daily basis suggested that cycling didn't increase acute pain in either of the groups.

What causes osteoarthritis patients to shed weight?

An overweight person suffering from knee OA was at a higher risk of the progression of structural change in the knee, and an increased likelihood for developing OA within the knee.

The significant relationship between small changes in the body mass index as well as the incidence of knee OA have been documented repeatedly. The findings in studies like the Framingham Heart study and the first National Health and Nutrition Examination Survey (NHANES I) revealed that those who had the most body weight had the highest chance for getting knee OA. Studies on prospective studies have also shown that those who are obese or overweight have significantly higher chance to develop knee OA and that weight loss dramatically lowers the risk of the development of knee OA(Focht).

Limitation of activity to OA knee sufferer

Certain activities could increase the rate of degenerative processes in OA knee. It is advised to avoid those actions.

These actions are

1. Squatting.

2. Legs crossed and sitting.

3. Stair climbing.

***

Late stage OA knee

The final stage is a severe stage that seriously affects the mobility of those suffering and they could even become bedridden. The knee appears swollen, and in a straight line becomes difficult. The severity of this condition can be seen clearly in the X-ray image.

The joint space between bones gets drastically reduced. The articular surface gets rough, and cartilage is nearly entirely gone. The synovial fluid has decreased significantly and does not help reduce the friction between the moving joints.

In these cases the knee is suggested. I have witnessed a dramatic transformation within the life of patients who have had the replacement procedure.

There are two types of surgery for replacement, namely a complete knee replacement (TKR) as well as a partially knee replacement (PKR). The surgeon makes the decision on the type of surgery that best fulfills your needs based on the degree of degeneration in your articular cartilage. Though, research reveals that PKR is as effective TKR and is also cost-effective(David).

Figure 35 The Total Knee Replacement

What exercises can be helpful at this point?

The reason for exercises at these stages is to get knee joints ready for surgery. A strong and healthy muscle is essential before surgery to prevent complications following surgery.

It determines how quickly and more effectively your recovery from the surgery is. The most serious post-surgical complication is muscle atrophy that affects your walk (walking patterns). Exercises can prevent this problem Also, exercises increase circulation of blood around the knee, which is crucial for the healing process after surgery.

Exercises during the late stage

Except for exercises that require land you can do all the exercises that we've discussed in the previous paragraphs.

Let me make reference to those exercises. For additional details about exercises, you can go back to the relevant chapters.

1. Static quadriceps exercise.

2. Dynamic quadriceps exercise.

3. Exercise to strengthen the adductor.

4. Exercise for strengthening the abductor.

5. Short abductor strengthening exercises.

Following the procedure after the procedure, exercise can be started from the day after surgery. There are several sets of exercises you have to do following replacement surgery which is known as the postoperative exercise regimen.

This is a crucial step in minimizing issues, encourages healing, and impacts the way you walk. The postoperative treatment protocol is beyond that of the subject matter in this guide.

Conclusion

Our knees are crucial and need to be properly taken care of since they give support and stability to our body. They also allow that our knees can straighten and bend which allows the user to walk or jog jump, run as well as climb up and down and turn. The knees consist of cartilage, bones, ligaments, muscles and tendon. Any injury to one of these could cause inflammation and pain. The knee pain is a possibility for all people regardless of their age, background, or race. There are numerous ways to treat knee pain at home like those discussed above that can be extremely beneficial for relieving pain in the knee however, in the case of extreme cases, it is advised to speak with the doctor for an in-depth examination. The knee pain can be experienced in a variety of knee structures. If you suffer from an infection, you'll not only feel pain but your knee could also get swollen and red. The degree of knee pain is different. A few may only experience an occasional ache, while others might experience pain that prevents the knee from performing any task.

There are many home remedies that you can do at home to alleviate knee pain. There are many other tips you can use to decrease the chance of injury in the knees. By following the advice that were mentioned earlier and working out regularly, you will strengthen your knees, reduce the chance of injury and discover a method to treat your knee discomfort.

www.ingramcontent.com/pod-product-compliance
Lightning Source LLC
Chambersburg PA
CBHW060330030426
42336CB00011B/1272